MW01223721

Connie W. Bales is Associate Director of the Sarah W. Stedman Center for Nutritional Studies, Associate Professor of Medicine, and Senior Fellow at the Center for the Study of Aging and Human Development at Duke University Medical Center. She holds a doctorate in Nutritional Science and is also a Registered Dietician.

Mark N. Feinglos is Professor of Medicine in the Division of Endocrinology, Metabolism and Nutrition; Associate Professor of Psychiatry and Behavioral Sciences; and Medical Director of Clinical Chemistry at Duke University Medical Center. His primary research interests involve the nutritional causes of type II diabetes and the dietary and pharmacological treatment of diabetes.

Claudia S. Plaisted is a nutrition writer and Registered and Licensed Dietitian with a master's degree in Clinical Nutrition and a background in psychology. She writes a nutrition column in the Southeastern regional magazine *Carolina Woman,* conducts research, counsels patients, and teaches Stopping the Diet Cycle, a group for the treatment of compulsive eating and weight cycling at the Stedman Center.

**Dietary Approaches to Healthy Living
from
The Sarah W. Stedman Center
for Nutritional Studies at
Duke University Medical Center**

Eating Well, Living Well with Hypertension
Eating Well, Living Well with Kidney Disease
Eating Well, Living Well with Osteoporosis

EATING WELL, LIVING WELL
with
DIABETES

Mark N. Feinglos, M.D., C.M.
Claudia S. Plaisted, M.S., R.D., L.D.N.

Connie W. Bales, PH.D., R.D.
Series Editor

with Linda J. Lumsden, PH.D., M.A.

VIKING

VIKING
Published by the Penguin Group
Penguin Books USA Inc., 375 Hudson Street,
New York, New York 10014, U.S.A.
Penguin Books Ltd, 27 Wrights Lane,
London W8 5TZ, England
Penguin Books Australia Ltd, Ringwood,
Victoria, Australia
Penguin Books Canada Ltd, 10 Alcorn Avenue,
Toronto, Ontario, Canada M4V 3B2
Penguin Books (N.Z.) Ltd, 182–190 Wairau Road,
Auckland 10, New Zealand

Penguin Books Ltd, Registered Offices:
Harmondsworth, Middlesex, England

First published in 1997 by Viking Penguin,
a division of Penguin Books USA Inc.

10 9 8 7 6 5 4 3 2 1

PUBLISHER'S NOTE
The ideas, procedures, and suggestions contained in this book are not
intended as a substitute for consulting with your physician. All matters
regarding your health require medical supervision.

LIBRARY OF CONGRESS CATALOGING-IN-PUBLICATION DATA
Feinglos, Mark N.
    Eating well, living well with diabetes / by Mark N. Feinglos and
Claudia S. Plaisted, with Linda J. Lumsden.
        p.   cm.
    "Dietary approaches to healthy living from the Sarah W. Stedman
Center for Nutritional Studies at Duke University Medical Center."
    Includes bibliographical references and index.
    ISBN 0-670-86657-1
    1. Diabetes—Diet therapy—Recipes.   2. Diabetes—Nutritional
aspects.   3. Diabetes—Popular works.   I. Plaisted, Claudia S.
II. Lumsden, Linda J.   III. Duke University.   Sarah W. Stedman
Center for Nutritional Studies.   IV. Title.
RC662.F45   1997
616.4′620654—dc20   96–27914

This book is printed on acid-free paper.

∞

Printed in the United States of America
Set in Minion

Contents

Foreword

ood nutrition is the cornerstone of good health. At the Sarah W. Stedman Center for Nutritional Studies, we are committed to the idea that optimum health care includes comprehensive nutritional care. At the Nutrition Center, we routinely incorporate the results of research studies on nutrition and disease into the medical/health care plans of our patients.

The purpose of the *Eating Well, Living Well* series is to share the expert knowledge of the medical doctors and nutritionists who work within the Duke Medical Center community at the level of nutritional therapy and lifestyle intervention. Education is the key to the prevention and treatment of many common diseases. Yet much of the information available today about nutrition and diet is incomplete or inaccurate. We hope that the *Eating Well, Living Well* series will begin to resolve some of the controversies associated with present-day diets.

Many popularly promoted diets are not founded on sound nutritional principles and common sense. Such diets are difficult for most people to follow, usually because there is no consideration for those with special health concerns. That is why we include in each book sections on selecting the right foods in a variety of settings, including grocery stores, restaurants, and recreational events. Another problem with catchall and fad diets is that there are often no special considerations for individual differences in activity, age, or lifestyle.

The *Eating Well, Living Well* series addresses these issues directly. We have asked experts from specific fields of clinical research and practice to write about disease prevention by nutritional means, with specific emphasis on individual differences and exceptions to the rules. Each book is uniquely tailored to each disease. This book explores the latest nutritional aspects of diabetes, a disease of metabolism and blood-glucose control that in the long term can lead to damage of sensitive organs of the body.

Sarah White Stedman

Chapter One

What Is Diabetes?

Believe it or not, a diagnosis of diabetes can be an invitation to a better life. Although the list of problems associated with diabetes is long and frightening, we now know that most, if not all, problems can be delayed or avoided through diet, exercise, and appropriate medication. The best defense against developing diabetes is to control your weight and stay active. The key to managing most cases of diabetes is to balance your diet, reduce fat intake, maintain a healthy weight, and keep your blood pressure normal for your entire life. These strategies help control blood-sugar levels, which clearly reduces the risk of diabetes complications.

Although the discovery of insulin in 1921 and other advances in treatment have made it possible for people with diabetes to live long and productive lives, the complications resulting from years of diabetes are responsible for considerable physical and financial hardship. Diabetes is the most common metabolic disease in the world, afflicting more than 100 million people; 14 million are Americans. Problems related to diabetes are responsible for one out of every seven dollars spent on health care in the United States. The disease is the fourth-leading cause of death in the United States, with more than 160,000 Americans dying annually from problems related to diabetes. Diabetic eye disease is the leading cause of blindness in adults and diabetic kidney disease the top cause of kidney failure. Nerve and circulation problems related to diabetes, as well as an increased rate of infection among diabetics, result in diabetes being a leading cause of foot and leg amputations. Diabetes doubles the odds that a person will suffer a heart attack or stroke. We now know, however, that these statistics can be changed.

Defining Diabetes

Diabetes is a metabolic disease, meaning it impairs the body's ability to burn the fuel it gets from food. The fuel is a simple sugar called *glucose*. Glucose provides the body with energy. Most of the food we eat is converted into glucose in the digestive tract. Glucose is absorbed into the bloodstream through the walls of the small intestine. Blood carries glucose to the cells, which convert it into energy. Glucose is to your body what gasoline is to your automobile. One way to think of diabetes is as a fuel distribution problem.

Normally, after eating, a rise in blood glucose triggers the pancreas to send *insulin* throughout your body. Insulin is a string of 51 amino acids that is produced by clusters of cells in the pancreas. Insulin signals trillions of cells in your body to open up to receive glucose.

A person with diabetes either does not make insulin naturally, does not make enough insulin, or is insensitive to the insulin that is made. Decreased production of insulin results from damage to the pancreatic cells. *Insulin resistance* is a result of the body's cells failing to understand insulin's signal to open up to receive the glucose. Without insulin, or the correct signal from insulin, glucose cannot get into the body's cells, so it forms a type of "logjam" in the blood. In turn, the cells of the pancreas can be poisoned by high blood-glucose levels, causing them to produce less insulin.

People with diabetes may also have high blood-fat levels, which are associated with heart disease, partly as a result of high glucose and low insulin. Over time, high blood-glucose levels combined with high blood-fat levels take a toll on other parts of the body, leading to the many complications that make diabetes so dangerous.

Types of Diabetes

About 5 to 10 percent of people with diabetes in the United States have *insulin-dependent diabetes mellitus (IDDM)*, or type I diabetes. This used to be called juvenile-onset diabetes because it often appears in children or young adults. They lose the ability to produce insulin because of autoimmune destruction of the pancreatic beta cells. The reason the body destroys these cells is not clear, but there is a genetic link.

People with IDDM always need insulin treatment to survive. Symptoms of IDDM often appear suddenly and may include extreme thirst, insatiable hunger, blurry vision, frequent urination, extreme fatigue, nausea, and unexplained weight loss.

The far more common form of diabetes is *non-insulin-dependent diabetes mellitus (NIDDM)*, also known as type II. This used to be called adult-onset diabetes. NIDDM affects about 90 percent of people with diabetes. It is found in 6.6 percent of all Americans between the ages of 20 and 74. In NIDDM, the insulin-producing cells in the pancreas make some insulin but not enough to function optimally. The insulin shortage causes blood glucose to build up.

The reason there is not enough insulin is that many people with NIDDM also are insulin resistant. That means the cells are unable to respond to the insulin signal, so blood glucose builds up despite the presence of insulin. The pancreas tries to secrete even more insulin, but the amount, although large for someone without diabetes, is not enough to move the blood glucose into the cells normally. Furthermore, the high insulin level is thought to raise the risk of heart disease. Insulin resistance and high insulin levels are also associated with high blood pressure and high blood-fat levels.

Symptoms of NIDDM are often much more subtle than those of IDDM but may include some fatigue and frequent thirst and urination. More than half the people who have NIDDM are unaware of it. The long-term problems of NIDDM are the same as those of IDDM. Of particular importance, people with NIDDM are at greater risk for circulation problems, stroke, and heart disease as a result of chronic damage to their large blood vessels. Although little direct proof exists, we think this is related to years of high blood glucose.

Only about a third of people with NIDDM need injections of insulin. Another third can manage the disease through diet, exercise, and pills that lower blood sugar, while the remaining third can manage the disease through diet and exercise alone. It may be that many people with NIDDM who take insulin could be treated without insulin if they followed a diet and exercise plan carefully.

People who are obese are more likely to develop NIDDM. More than 80 percent of people with NIDDM are 20 percent or more over their recommended weight. NIDDM often can be avoided by eating well and exercising regularly. In contrast, IDDM so far cannot be prevented. Diet, exercise, and tight blood-glucose control, however, can delay or minimize complications.

A third form of diabetes is gestational diabetes, which occurs among 3 to 4 percent of all pregnant women—some 90,000 women annually. Pregnant women should be screened for diabetes between the 24th and 28th week of pregnancy. Gestational diabetes usually goes away after pregnancy, but about half these women will develop permanent diabetes in 10 to 20 years. Diabetic women who become pregnant are more vulnerable to obstetrical complications. It is imperative that they seek prenatal care early in their pregnancy to help ensure a smooth pregnancy and delivery.

Finally, some people may develop diabetes as a complication of another disease. A severe inflammation of the pancreas, for example, can cause diabetes, as can the prolonged use of high doses of corticosteroid drugs such as Prednisone.

Who Is at Risk for NIDDM?

Diabetes is a disease that has both genetic and environmental causes. If either of your parents was diagnosed with NIDDM after age 50, the chances are one in thirteen that you will inherit the disease. The odds increase to one in seven if either parent was diagnosed before age 50, and they approach one in two in families with very early onset (in the teens and twenties) of NIDDM. If both of your parents have NIDDM, your chances of developing diabetes are 50 percent.

NIDDM occurs more frequently among certain ethnic groups, including African Americans, Hispanic Americans, and Native Americans. Diabetes is 16 percent more common among African American men than Caucasian men, for instance, and is 50 percent more common among African-American women than Caucasian women.

The complications of diabetes often take a greater toll on minorities, perhaps because of socioeconomic and lifestyle factors, but also because of genetic factors. Hispanic Americans, for instance, are more likely to experience two specific complications from their diabetes: kidney disease (three to five times) and retinopathy (two to three times), the leading cause of blindness in the nation.

Diagnosing Diabetes

If you suspect you have diabetes or are at risk for the disease, make an appointment with your physician. You can expect him or her to take a complete medical history and give you a complete physical examination. The physician will conduct several blood and urine tests to measure your blood glucose, hemoglobin, and cholesterol, and test for protein in your urine.

The most common diagnostic test is the *fasting plasma glucose test*. If you are going to have this test done, you must not eat or drink anything except water after midnight before the test. In the morning you will visit a laboratory, where a technician will take a blood sample. A blood-glucose reading greater than 140 milligrams per deciliter (140 mg/dl) on two separate occasions indicates diabetes. A normal fasting plasma glucose reading is between about 70 mg/dl and 115 mg/dl. Readings between 115 mg/dl and 140 mg/dl are defined as impaired glucose tolerance. One third to one half the people with impaired glucose tolerance will ultimately develop diabetes.

The *oral glucose tolerance test* is another diagnostic tool. This test may be performed if information from the fasting glucose test is insufficient, if there are multiple risk factors for diabetes, or if you are pregnant. As with the fasting plasma glucose test, you must fast overnight before giving a blood sample. Then you will be asked to drink 75 grams of glucose. Your glucose level will be measured five times over three hours. A diabetes diagnosis follows if your glucose rises higher than 200 mg/dl two hours after drinking the glucose, even if your fasting glucose level is normal. A normal two-hour glucose value is about 70 to 140 mg/dl (higher in older people). Values between 140 mg/dl and 200 mg/dl are defined as impaired glucose tolerance.

Another useful test for diabetes is a *hemoglobin A1c* or *glycated hemoglobin (GHb) test*. Hemoglobin is the protein in red blood cells that carries oxygen. GHb forms when glucose in the blood attaches to the hemoglobin. The amount formed depends on the level of the blood glucose: higher blood-glucose levels mean higher levels of GHb. Since red blood cells stay in circulation an average of 120 days, the GHb level is a good measure of a person's average blood-glucose level over the past two to three months.

Urine tests for diabetes are unreliable, as glucose appears in the urine only when the blood glucose is over 180 (and in some people even higher). If blood testing is unavailable, a positive urine test is an indication that diabetes may be present.

People with IDDM are prone to a condition called *ketoacidosis*, which occurs when your body starts burning fat for energy because the cells can't get glucose from the blood. One byproduct of burning fat is *ketones*. Ketoacidosis occurs when too many ketones build up in the blood, and it means your diabetes is seriously out of control. In addition to experiencing symptoms of high blood glucose, persons with ketoacidosis may experience nausea, vomiting, rapid breathing, or loss of consciousness.

Some 75,000 people in the United States are hospitalized annually with ketoacidosis; 4,000 of them die. People with IDDM who have very high blood-glucose levels or are ill regardless of blood-glucose levels should test their urine for ketones. Your doctor will show you how to do this. It is extremely unusual for people with NIDDM to develop ketoacidosis, but it can occur sometimes with very serious illness.

Your Diabetes Care Team

You are the most important member of your diabetes care team. Other members should include a physician, a diabetes educator, a registered dietitian, and a pharmacist. Your diabetes physician may be a family practitioner, a general internist, or an endocrinologist. If your primary-care physician has no special program for people with diabetes, he or she can refer you to a diabetes teaching program or an endocrinologist.

A counselor or other mental health professional who can offer you emotional support should also be available, because stress can raise blood glucose. Learning how to cope with emotional stresses can help you control your diabetes. You need to be able to vent your concerns and feelings in a safe place. A counselor may help you and your spouse or others close to you to open up and share these feelings. A diabetes support group may be another valuable resource for you. One benefit reported by some people diagnosed with diabetes, incidentally, is improved communication and closeness with their family.

Experts agree that diet is the cornerstone of diabetes treatment. For most people it is the single most important factor in managing their diabetes. A dietitian or nutritionist therefore can play an important part in your health care team. In the United States, about 30 percent of people with diabetes are treated with dietary measures alone, usually in association with an exercise program. A diet for someone with diabetes is virtually the same as one that any expert would prescribe for anyone who wants to live a long and healthy life. By following commonsense diet recommendations for diabetes you will lower your risk for heart disease, kidney disease, and some forms of cancer. By exercising regularly you will be stronger, leaner, and more energetic.

The positive aspect of most diabetes is that you can control almost all the factors that trigger or exacerbate the disease. The best reason for you to take charge of your diabetes is that it is much easier to control diabetes than it is to deal with the many serious complications the disease can cause.

You will recognize other benefits of a diabetes diagnosis as you begin to eat more healthfully and become more active. Remember that the single most important member of your diabetes team is you. You possess the power not only to control your diabetes but to become healthier—and happier—through diet, exercise, and tight blood-glucose management. Chapter Two will discuss these three components of successful diabetes management.

Chapter Two

Treating Diabetes

D iet, exercise, and medication form the foundation of treatment for diabetes. Diabetes management seeks to maintain a proper balance between glucose and insulin. The guiding principle is that food (or not enough insulin) raises the blood-glucose level, and medication and exercise lower it.

The role that diet, exercise, and medication play in keeping glucose under tight control was underscored by the results of the Diabetes Control and Complications Trial (DCCT), a 10-year trial of 1,400 IDDM patients that ended in June 1993. This landmark study concluded that keeping tight control of blood glucose through diet and medication is the key to reducing complications from diabetes. It strongly pointed to elevated blood glucose as the cause of long-term diabetic complications. Complications in subjects who kept tight control of their blood glucose were substantially lowered in the DCCT. Compared with less intensive therapy, some of the results included the following:

- a 76-percent decrease in the risk of developing retinopathy (disease of the retina of the eye)
- a 54-percent decrease in the progression of diabetic retinopathy
- a 60-percent decrease in clinical neuropathy (nerve disease)
- a 54-percent decrease in the risk of developing clinical albuminuria, which is an early marker for nephropathy (kidney disease)

The DCCT found that lifestyle changes had the most impact upon maintaining tight control over blood-glucose levels. These changes included the following:

- monitoring blood glucose regularly
- exercising regularly
- administering insulin as needed
- visiting health professionals on a regular basis
- maintaining a meal plan with the help of a diabetes care team

Blood-Glucose Monitoring

People in the DCCT who were most successful in keeping their diabetes under control tested their glucose four times a day. Normal blood-glucose readings are between 70 and 115 mg/dl before breakfast and 70 to 140 mg/dl before other meals. In reality, absolutely normal values cannot routinely be achieved without episodes of low blood glucose, or *hypoglycemia*. The goal is to get as close to normal as is reasonable, and that level can vary from person to person.

It is important to keep a good record of your glucose so you can tell how effectively you are keeping your diabetes in check and whether you need to make any adjustments in your diabetes care plan. Initially after receiving a diabetes diagnosis, you should test your blood glucose four or more times per day until you establish the correct balance of insulin and glucose. Try doing measurements before eating and then two hours after to see how your body reacts to different foods. You should also record any unusual circumstances that may affect your glucose reading, such as a stressful event or schedule change. Once your blood-glucose level is stabilized, you should continue to test your blood glucose up to four times daily. The best time to test is before breakfast, lunch, and dinner and at bedtime, or two hours after meals. Some people benefit from periodically checking between 2:00 and 3:00 A.M.

To test your blood-glucose level, you need a drop of blood pricked with a special lancet or a small automated device. The machine is so fast it makes obtaining blood from your finger almost painless. Keep an accurate and consistent record of your blood-glucose levels. The record will help you learn over time what triggers high and low blood-glucose readings. Bring your blood-glucose record to your meetings with your diabetes care team so you can get their expert advice on how to improve your blood-glucose levels. Your team can help you make changes in your lifestyle and come up with strategies to avoid blood-glucose fluctuations.

Diet

Diet plays the biggest role in managing NIDDM. While people with IDDM will always require insulin, changing one's diet can enable many people with NIDDM to reduce the amount of insulin or other diabetes medication they need.

Since 1994, the American Diabetes Association (ADA)

Nutrition Recommendations for People with Diabetes Mellitus have emphasized differences among people by individualizing meal plans. The new guidelines call for liberalizing previous limitations on sugar and focusing on total carbohydrates as opposed to the sources of those carbohydrates. Generally, they call for eating less fat, a variety of fresh vegetables and fruit, fewer sugary foods, and lean meat and fish.

The new ADA guidelines are similar to the general Dietary Guidelines for Americans issued in recent years by the U.S. Departments of Agriculture and Health and Human Services, as well as recommendations by the American Heart Association and the American Cancer Society.

Weight loss is often an important component of diet management for diabetes, since 85 percent of people with NIDDM are at least 20 percent overweight, and obesity is a major risk factor for developing diabetes. Another compelling reason for people with diabetes to treat obesity is that losing weight increases insulin sensitivity and thus reduces the body's need for insulin. Some people with NIDDM may even be able to stop using insulin after losing weight. Even a loss of 5 to 10 pounds can result in improved blood pressure and lowered levels of blood glucose and blood fat. Since reducing fat intake helps people lose weight, overweight people with diabetes or at risk for the disease should pay special attention to that portion of their diet.

Fat causes special problems for people with diabetes. Most Americans eat too much fat, sugar, and sodium (salt). Nearly two of every three calories consumed by the average American comes from fat or sugar. These substances are not particularly good for anyone, but they are especially unhealthy for people with diabetes. People with diabetes are at higher risk for obesity, hypertension, and high cholesterol—all conditions associated with fat that contribute to heart disease. An important component of changing your diet will be to reduce the amount of fat you consume.

The new emphasis upon individualizing diets means you have more responsibility for and control over creating a diabetes meal plan that works for you. You need to decide what, when, and how much you will eat throughout the day to meet your daily nutritional needs while keeping your blood-glucose levels in control. Working with your dietitian, you should develop a plan that fits your lifestyle, food tastes, budget, schedule, and medical needs. You will need to learn not only about food plans but about dietary fat, cholesterol, and perhaps food exchanges to keep your diabetes under control. See Chapter Five for specific recommendations on how to create a meal plan to manage your diabetes.

Exercise

Exercise is another way to reduce the negative effects of diabetes. Exercise helps move glucose from the blood to the muscle cells, maintains fitness, helps normalize blood-glucose levels, reduces stress, and helps control weight. Exercise will not only help you lose weight but will help you keep that weight off.

When you exercise, your muscles move more blood glucose into the cells. The muscle cells also become more insulin sensitive, meaning they will use insulin more efficiently and probably require less medication. The body remains more sensitive to insulin from 24 to 48 hours after the exercise stops.

The type of exercise program you choose need not be complicated or expensive. Walking, for instance, is as beneficial as it is simple. The most important criterion for your exercise program is that you choose an activity you enjoy so that you will stick with it. Try to find a partner to join you for walks, bicycle rides, swimming, or tennis to make exercise more enjoyable.

Before you embark upon an exercise program, you should ask your doctor for advice on what kinds of exercise are appropriate for you, especially if you are not used to exercising regularly. If you have heart disease, high cholesterol, or smoke cigarettes, you should take an exercise test while hooked up to an EKG machine to see how your heart responds. If you have complications from diabetes such as kidney problems or retinopathy, you should also ask your doctor how those conditions will affect your exercise program. If you have IDDM and your blood glucose is above 250 mg/dl, check your blood glucose and urine for ketones before and after you exercise. Vigorous exercise can sometimes make glucose control deteriorate in people with poorly controlled IDDM.

If you use insulin or oral agents to help control your diabetes, you should consider checking your blood glucose before and after exercise on a few occasions to see how the activity affects your blood-glucose level. If your blood glucose drops too low during exercise, you will need to take steps to correct it. Discuss this with your physician before you head to the gym the first time.

You will probably notice a difference in your glucose levels within a few weeks after embarking upon your exercise program. Besides helping you look trimmer and feel more energetic, exercise may lower your glucose level to the point where you can reduce or even eliminate (if you have NIDDM) your insulin dose.

Stress and Diabetes

Stress and mood will affect your diabetes. Stress makes blood glucose rise when "fight or flight" hormones release energy from glucose and fat. A fight with your boss or a long line at the supermarket checkout counter can translate into elevated glucose.

Coping with diabetes may add stress to your life. Diabetes is a complicated disease, and the sudden entrance into your life of daily blood tests and medication, regular visits to the doctor, and the potential for serious complications is stressful, to say the least. High blood glucose itself can make you feel fatigued and "down."

No one can eliminate all stress from his or her life, but we can all find ways to reduce stress. A daily walk or swim gives you some quiet time and a physical outlet for frustration. A jazzercise or karate class may offer you a relaxing social outlet as well as a physical workout.

Meditation can also alleviate stress. Meditation and related relaxation techniques have been shown to reduce pulse rate and blood pressure, both of which are physical indicators of stress. A professional may be able to help you master relaxation techniques such as imaging, in which you imagine soothing scenes, or biofeedback, in which you learn to consciously relax muscles. Studies have shown that all of these techniques can lower blood glucose.

For some people, successful stress management may begin with saying no to requests and demands upon your time. This may become important as you come to terms with managing a chronic disease. Sometimes settling into bed with a good book or treating yourself to a matinee movie gives you a sufficient break from your responsibilities to relax and reduce stress. The key to reducing stress is to find an enjoyable, safe activity that will make you feel good about yourself without doing harm to your body. These positive steps are healthy alternatives to harmful ways of handling stress, such as overeating, smoking cigarettes, or drinking excessive amounts of alcohol, all of which can aggravate diabetes.

Not everyone, however, can control his or her diabetes through diet and exercise alone. All people with IDDM (and some people with NIDDM) need insulin, regardless of how well they handle the other parts of their treatment plan. This is nothing to feel guilty about.

Medication

The idea of insulin injections makes some people nervous, but insulin plays an integral role in diabetes management. Before the discovery of insulin, most people with what we now call IDDM died within two years of diagnosis. Today, insulin makes it possible for millions of people with diabetes to live long and productive lives. Some 3 million Americans inject insulin daily to manage their diabetes in addition to diet and exercise therapy.

One crucial function of your diabetes team is for the appropriate member to teach you how to follow an insulin regimen and how to inject insulin. The team also can refer you to a diabetes education program that will cover this information. Hospitals and local diabetes information centers routinely offer such programs. Pharmacists also offer insulin instruction. After some instruction and practice, you will be able to administer insulin within a minute.

Many people with NIDDM can get along without insulin injections and need only take oral antidiabetic agents to boost the insulin output from their pancreas or to make their body more sensitive to insulin.

You must monitor your blood glucose especially closely for two to four weeks after beginning therapy with oral agents to make sure you are taking the appropriate dose. Elderly people should be cautious about using *sulfonylureas,* pills that both boost the pancreas's production of insulin and improve insulin sensitivity. And people with liver or kidney disease should never use them, because decreased kidney or liver function may make it difficult for your body to process the drug correctly. High levels may build up and cause *hypoglycemia.*

Hypoglycemia

Hypoglycemia occurs when blood-glucose levels drop too low. Medications that keep blood glucose in check also can put you at risk for hypoglycemia. Also called an *insulin reaction,* hypoglycemia can occur if you take too much insulin (or oral medication) or fail to eat enough food. A hypoglycemic attack is most likely to occur just before a meal, when glucose levels are lowest; at the peak time of the insulin; and during or shortly after exercise.

Hypoglycemia can be serious. Early symptoms may include sweating, pallor, blurry vision, a clammy feeling, dizziness, a confused state, hunger, irritability, personality change, shaking, headache, drowsiness, poor coordination, and a rapid pulse. An extremely low blood-glucose level can result in unconsciousness, seizures, or even death.

Anyone suffering a hypoglycemic attack needs to eat some glucose immediately. One-third cup of orange juice or regular soda (not diet soda) or two glucose tablets should be sufficient to relieve the symptoms. Drink or eat the substance again if symptoms do not go away in 15 minutes. If they persist, go to the emergency room. Don't eat anything with lots of fat in it, such as a candy bar, as fat slows the absorption of glucose into the bloodstream.

People who use insulin are especially vulnerable to a drop in blood glucose when they exercise. To avoid hypoglycemia, eat a high-carbohydrate snack, such as an apple or a banana, within the hour previous to the physical activity. Wait at least 45 to 60 minutes after injecting insulin to exercise, because insulin absorption from the injection site may be enhanced soon after the injection, dropping your glucose level. Do not go to sleep after exercising without eating. Hypoglycemia is a special risk during the middle of the night. A low-fat snack before bedtime greatly reduces the possibility of a hypoglycemic attack during the night.

Chapter Three

Nutrition and Diabetes

A healthy diet for a person with diabetes is just like a healthy diet for anyone: a balanced diet that features a variety of foods to provide you with the right amount of carbohydrate, protein, and fat, as well as fiber, vitamins, and minerals. The other nutritional goals for people with diabetes are to maintain appropriate blood-glucose and blood-fat levels, to maintain a reasonable body weight, and to eat meals and snacks consistently to maximize blood-glucose control.

The Bottom Line: Where Calories Come From

Good nutrition means eating the correct balance of foods. Your body can get calories from only four classes of foods: carbohydrates, proteins, fats, and alcohol. Your body requires insulin to use the glucose form of energy from all of these foods.

Carbohydrates should make up the bulk of your diet because they give your body most of its energy. They give your body 4 calories of energy for every gram. Carbohydrates come in two forms, sugars and starches. Sugars are simple carbohydrates. They are found naturally in fruits and their juices and are added in refined form to many foods, such as soda and cookies. Starches are complex carbohydrates and are found in pastas, cereals, breads, legumes (beans and peas), and vegetables. Foods that are mostly complex carbohydrate are often good sources of fiber, too. These include whole-grain foods, legumes, vegetables, and the simple carbohydrate, fruit.

Protein is an essential part of the diet that builds most of our muscles, blood cells, skin, and hair. Like carbohydrates, it provides 4 calories for every gram. Protein is found in meat, fish, milk, cheese, and eggs, and to a lesser extent in plants such as legumes, grains, and vegetables. Up to 20 percent of your daily calories should come from protein. People with kidney disease, a complication of diabetes, benefit from eating less protein and should consult a registered dietitian or licensed nutritionist to work on their special dietary needs. While protein is essential, Americans generally consume too much animal-based protein, which is often high in fat.

Fat is a concentrated form of energy that your body needs in order to work well, but fat must be consumed sparingly, since it is very rich in calories: there are 9 calories in every gram of fat you eat. Fat is found in meats, dairy products, oils, nuts, and spreads such as butter and margarine, and baked goods. Fat is the culprit behind so many health problems for people with diabetes that all of Chapter Four is devoted to fats and weight management. Eating too much fat can raise your risk for heart disease, the leading cause of death not only among people with diabetes but among all Americans. Diets high in fat can also contribute to obesity.

Alcohol gives your body 7 calories in every gram, and virtually nothing else. It contains practically no vitamins or minerals. Therefore, it is an added source of empty calories. Many people with diabetes find that consuming alcohol interferes with their diabetes management. Before you decide to include alcohol in your diet, consult your physician.

Insulin: How Glucose Gets Around

Insulin plays a starring role in helping your body to use these nutrients after they turn into glucose, your body's source of fuel. Virtually all of carbohydrate ends up as glucose, and more than half of protein turns into glucose. Fat is different. While it has little direct effect on blood glucose, its indirect effect can be profound, as too much dietary fat is a risk factor for obesity, which itself is a risk factor for diabetes. Each of these types of energy sources has a different effect upon your blood-glucose levels.

The Food Guide Pyramid

The most up-to-date guidelines for eating a healthy, balanced diet are found in the Food Guide Pyramid created in 1992 by the U.S. Department of Agriculture (USDA) and the U.S. Department of Health and Human Services and modified for the special concerns of diabetes by the American Diabetes Association. The Stedman Center recommends that anyone with diabetes follow the ADA Food Guide Pyramid's recommendations for all Americans. The pyramid replaces the Basic Four Food Groups you might have learned about in school. The new Food Guide Pyramid calls for less fat and meat and many more fruits, vegetables, and grain products in the American diet than the old Basic Four plan.

The new pyramid makes it easier to visualize how different kinds of foods fit into a healthy diet. It divides foods into six groups: breads and other starches, vegetables, fruits, protein, dairy, and fats, oils, and sugars. The idea behind the pyramid is that anyone who eats the minimum recommended amount of foods from the first five groups every day will probably receive adequate amounts of the more than 50 nutrients identified as essential to human health.

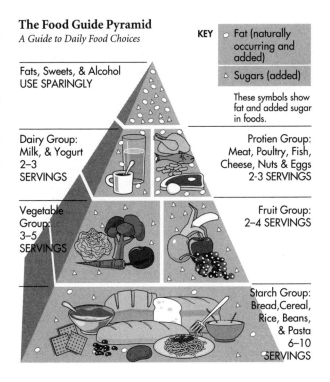

The Food Guide Pyramid
A Guide to Daily Food Choices

KEY
○ Fat (naturally occurring and added)
△ Sugars (added)

These symbols show fat and added sugar in foods.

Fats, Sweets, & Alcohol
USE SPARINGLY

Dairy Group:
Milk, & Yogurt
2–3
SERVINGS

Protien Group:
Meat, Poultry, Fish,
Cheese, Nuts & Eggs
2-3 SERVINGS

Vegetable
Group:
3–5
SERVINGS

Fruit Group:
2–4 SERVINGS

Starch Group:
Bread,Cereal,
Rice, Beans,
& Pasta
6–10
SERVINGS

Bread, cereal, rice, beans, and pasta compose the bottom of the pyramid and its largest part, and they should serve as the foundation of your daily diet. These foods supply most of our carbohydrates, thiamin, iron, and niacin.

Whole-grain products are also good sources of fiber. You should eat *at least* six to ten servings a day from this group—and you may need even more depending on your age, height, weight, and activity level. A serving from this group equals one slice of bread, about three-fourths cup of cereal, one-half cup of cooked beans, or one-half cup of cooked pasta or rice.

The second tier of the pyramid houses vegetables and fruits. These are our major sources of vitamins A and C, as well as fiber, which aids digestion. You should eat at least three servings of vegetables a day, although up to five or more servings are recommended. A serving equals a cup of raw leafy vegetables, three-quarters of a cup of vegetable juice, or half a cup of cooked vegetables. You should also eat two to four servings of fruit a day. A serving equals one medium raw fruit, one-half cup of fruit juice, or half a cup of cooked or canned fruit.

The third tier comprises the dairy and protein groups. Red meats, fish, poultry and cheese substitutes are major sources of protein, niacin, iron, and thiamin. You should eat two to three servings of protein daily. One serving of protein equals 2 to 3 ounces of cooked lean meat, fish, or poultry; two eggs; or 2 ounces of low-fat cheese. A healthy, low-fat diet that is adequate in protein requires only about 6 ounces of protein a day. Visually, that is about the size of two decks of cards a day of meat, fish, or poultry. If you are eating three or four decks' worth, then you may be eating too much protein—and too much fat, saturated fat, and cholesterol.

Milk products supply protein, vitamin D, phosphorus, potassium, thiamin, and, most important, 76 percent of our calcium. At the very least, you should eat two servings from the dairy group daily, and for many people three servings is preferable. If you are at risk for osteoporosis, you might want to work three dairy servings into your meal plan. One serving from the dairy group equals a cup of milk or regular yogurt. (You should treat one-third cup of frozen yogurt as one bread serving.)

Butter, margarine, sour cream, oil, shortening, and sugar are a part of the pyramid's narrow tip and are sprinkled sparsely throughout its remainder. Use fats, oils, and sugars sparingly. The different types of fat and how they affect your health are explained in Chapter Four.

The new nutritional recommendations also call for people to consume 20 to 30 grams of fiber daily. Most Americans consume only a fraction of that amount. *Fiber* is the part of plant foods that you cannot digest, and it passes through your body largely unchanged. Fiber adds bulk to your diet and helps you to eliminate waste. There are two types of fiber. *Insoluble fiber* is found in whole-wheat products and wheat bran and adds bulk for roughage. *Soluble fiber* is found in legumes, some fruits and vegetables, oat bran, and barley. It holds fluid to help keep the stool soft and more comfortable to pass. It also has been shown to lower blood cholesterol in some studies. Both types of fiber may play a role in reducing the risk of bowel cancer. Soluble fiber may help you control your blood glucose by slowing the absorption of food. These are all good reasons to get more fiber into your diet. Here are some tips on how to do it:

- Eat at least five servings of fruits and vegetables daily.
- Choose unrefined over refined grain products whenever possible, whole-grain breads and cereals (including oatmeal), brown rice, and unbuttered or plain popcorn.
- Eat a high-fiber bran cereal for breakfast.
- Add one-quarter cup miller's bran daily to foods such as cooked cereal, applesauce, and meat loaf.
- Eat cooked beans at least once a week.

ADA Guidelines

The Food Guide Pyramid is nearly identical to the 1994 American Diabetes Association Nutrition Recommendations for People with Diabetes Mellitus, which emphasize differences among people by individualizing meal plans. The new guidelines, which the Stedman Center also recommends, call for liberalizing previous limitations on sugar and focusing on total carbohydrates as opposed to the sources of those carbohydrates.

ADA recommendations for people with IDDM and NIDDM differ little. The biggest differences between meal plans have to do with age. Diets for children with IDDM, for instance, contain lots of calories so they can grow strong and healthy. Diets for teenagers emphasize flexibility, since youths in this age group are often on the go. Diets for adults call for lower fat and protein. Since most people with NIDDM are overweight, the ADA recommendations generally call for cutting 200 to 300 calories daily and exercising regularly to promote a healthy weight. The ADA suggests that people with NIDDM who are at a desirable weight spread out their caloric intake throughout the day. Otherwise, diet recommendations are the same.

The American Heart Association recommends that no more than 30 percent of your calories come from fat, with an emphasis on monounsaturated and polyunsaturated fats (this will be explained in Chapter Four). About 10 to 20 percent of calories typically come from protein. The remaining 60 to 70 percent should come from carbohydrates and fats, but the precise mix will vary depending on the relative importance to the individual of controlling blood glucose, blood fat, and weight. In treating individuals with diabetes, the Stedman Center diabetes care team follows the ADA guidelines because these recommendations are somewhat more flexible than the USDA

Dietary Guidelines for Americans. Other ADA diet recommendations follow the USDA guidelines. Here are some of the highlights.

Cholesterol
Limit cholesterol to no more than 300 milligrams daily. Nearly half of all Americans have blood-cholesterol levels above the recommended 200 mg/dl. High cholesterol is associated with heart disease, the leading cause of death among people with diabetes. See Chapter Four for more information on cholesterol.

Sodium
Sodium is usually eaten in the form of sodium chloride, most commonly known as table salt. Population studies suggest that diets high in sodium raise the risk for hypertension, or high blood pressure, which is more common in people with diabetes. Controlling high blood pressure is important if you have diabetes because it increases your risk for diabetic complications such as heart disease, kidney disease, eye problems, and strokes. Try to limit sodium to between 1,100 and 3,300 milligrams daily. People with mild to moderate hypertension should limit sodium to 2,200 milligrams daily.

Alcohol
Alcohol may cause blood glucose to drop in some people with diabetes using insulin or the oral medications called sulfonylureas. It also contains 7 calories per gram but virtually no nutrients, so it can easily pack on weight. But people who have their diabetes and weight under control may drink a moderate amount of alcohol, preferably with a meal if they take insulin. A moderate amount of alcohol is defined as one or two servings of 1 jigger (1¼ ounces) of hard liquor (approximately one cocktail), one 4-to-5-ounce glass of wine, or one 12-ounce can of beer. Al-

though you may have read about the alleged health benefits of moderate alcohol consumption, do not assume that adding it to your diet will enhance your risk factors until you speak with your diabetes care team. Check with your health care professional before including alcohol in your diet. And remember to include alcohol as part of your meal plan.

Vitamins and Minerals

Your body also needs vitamins and minerals for a healthy, balanced diet. The best sources of these are fruits and vegetables, whole-grain breads and cereals, and lean meats and low-fat dairy products—in other words, wholesome food.

Vitamins and some minerals work as enzymes and cofactors that help release energy but contain no energy themselves. You get no calories—and no direct energy—from these substances. Vitamin and mineral supplements have enjoyed immense popularity in recent years. While these products possess some health value, downing supplements is not the same as eating a balanced diet. Vitamin and mineral pills do not replace the nutrients found in vegetables and fruits, and recent research has shown that they do not possess their anti-cancer, anti-heart-disease benefits. It seems that there are other elements in food important for health—such as lignins, phytoestrogens, phytols, flavonoids, and fibers—that you can get only in fruits, vegetables, and legumes. The key to a healthy, balanced diet is to eat a moderate amount of a wide variety of foods that provide you with the proper proportion of the nutrients your body needs.

Artificial Sweeteners

Saccharin, aspartame, and acesulfame K are nonnutritive sweeteners approved by the FDA. They contain no calories. They are safe for people with diabetes to consume as an alternative to sugar.

The Scoop on Sugar

One of the biggest changes in the 1994 ADA recommendations is that table sugar is no longer forbidden. New research has shown that table sugar, or sucrose, does not cause blood-glucose levels to rise any more than other foods. Since nearly all food (except fat) turns into glucose, it doesn't matter what form food is in when you eat it: it still ends up as glucose. Although some debate continues among physicians and scientists, research suggests that how high your blood glucose rises after eating is more closely related to how much carbohydrate, not the kind of carbohydrate, you ate.

This rise in blood sugar is also related to your blood-glucose control. For example, if you keep your blood glucose tightly within the normal range, eating a small dessert after a meal is unlikely to have much effect on your glucose levels. However, if your blood glucose is poorly controlled and you eat dessert, you are much more likely to get high readings even two hours after your meal.

Different foods may affect your blood sugar differently. Blood-glucose monitoring before and after meals will help you determine how individual carbohydrate foods affect your glucose levels. Regardless of the effect on your blood glucose, however, plain table sugar has no vitamins or minerals in it, so nutritionally it is not a good choice.

But you should know that table sugar isn't the only simple sugar either naturally occurring or added to foods. Also look for dextrose, maltose, glucose, lactose, galactose, and fructose. They are easy to recognize on an ingredient label since they all end in "-ose."

In general, all sugars end up as glucose. Some people mistakenly believe that fructose is healthier than sucrose. This is not true for anyone, but for people with diabetes this misconception may be particularly harmful. Although limited amounts of fructose are unlikely to have any negative effect within the context of following your meal plan and eating a healthy diet, fructose is not a good choice to treat hypoglycemia (low blood glucose) because it can enter your muscle cells directly, leaving your brain without the glucose it so desperately needs. Remember that if you experience hypoglycemia, the best treatment is a glucose tablet or a source of sucrose that will give you 15 grams of carbohydrate. Orange juice, the old standby, works just fine, since many of its natural sugars are in the form of sucrose. Regular (not diet) soda can also be used. Although it contains a lot of fructose, a considerable amount of glucose is also present.

If any of these sugars are listed in the first three or four ingredients on the food label of a product you want to eat, take a second look. It may contain more sugar than is nutritionally sound.

The new view on sugars does not mean you can stop eating fruits and vegetables and dive into a box of table sugar. The problem with sugars is that they lack staying power because they are digested so quickly. Sugars cannot provide your body with fuel for very long. Nor can they provide fiber or significant minerals, vitamins, or nutrients. They can also cause dental cavities. If you are going to eat sugar, fit it into your meal plan as part of the total amount of carbohydrates for a particular meal or snack. Moderation is the key. It takes a balance of foods to make a healthy diet and a healthy person, not just tight glucose control.

The one item sugar provides in abundance is calories, and the only connection between diabetes and sugar is weight gain. There is no evidence that eating sugar actually causes diabetes. But when you start substituting three ginger snaps for a slice of bread, or a cup of frozen yogurt for a potato, you start adding a lot of fat and extra calories to your diet (and missing out on lots of healthy nutrients). There is evidence that dietary fat may play a role in developing NIDDM in predisposed animals and in at least some groups of humans. You can expect your blood glucose to rise when you eat 30 grams of carbohydrates whether it comes from an apple or a half cup of ice cream. But while that apple contains 120 calories, the ice cream packs 300 calories and is loaded with fat.

Sugars in whole foods are usually the healthiest choice because you're also consuming the other nutrients, vitamins, and fiber they contain. Whole foods include whole fruits (rather than fruit juices, punches, sodas, or fruited drinks such as sweetened iced teas), whole-grain breads and cereals, beans, peas, rice, pasta, and low-fat (1.5 percent or less) milk and milk products.

Much more than sugar, it is fat which is to blame for diabetes-related complications. Research suggests that many overweight people eat far more fat than sugar. Obesity puts people at great risk for developing diabetes, make diabetes harder to control, increases the risk for high blood pressure and heart disease, and interferes with the body's ability to use insulin effectively.

Chapter Four

Dietary Fat

Most people find that as their weight increases, their blood glucose also increases, and their diabetes becomes harder to control. Recent weight gain may explain why a person can have diabetes now but did not when he or she weighed less. In many cases, this process is reversible. Many people who are overweight and have NIDDM find that they can reduce or even stop their medications when they follow a healthy diet or lose weight.

Obesity and Overweight

When you gain excess weight, your body does not function at its peak level of performance. This is particularly true when it comes to how the hormone insulin works to control your blood glucose. As a person's weight goes up, the ability of his insulin to deliver glucose to the muscle cells goes down. This is often referred to as "insulin resistance" (see Chapter One).

When insulin works poorly and your blood-glucose

levels are high, your fat cells see the glucose as food available for storage. Unlike muscle cells, fat cells need very little insulin to pick up glucose, so the glucose feeds fat cells instead of muscle cells. Your muscle cells are starving while your fat cells are feasting. One negative consequence of this is that you must take larger doses of insulin or pills to enable glucose to enter your muscle cells. And gaining weight can cause your blood pressure to rise, too.

The best way to lose weight is gradually, so that it stays off permanently. Don't rely on fast, short-term gimmicks to help you manage your weight or your diabetes: they don't deliver what they promise. In addition, if you are taking medications, particularly insulin, you may provoke hypoglycemia attacks if you suddenly drop your caloric intake. Make sure you check with your physician and dietitian before you make any radical changes to your diet. Remember that small changes in your nutritional patterns, such as moderating fat content and making sensible food choices, can result in large improvements in your health.

Similarly, a small change in weight—even as little as 10 pounds—can lower your blood pressure and your fasting glucose level. In fact, the best plan for losing weight is to follow your meal plan, exercise regularly, and take your medications as prescribed. Since dietary fat plays such a large role in weight and health management, we will discuss it in some depth before looking at guidelines for successful weight loss while continuing to eat a balanced diet.

The Skinny on Fats

Many people find it challenging to understand fat and cholesterol. How does the fat and cholesterol on your plate differ from that in your bloodstream? First we will explain dietary fats, which are the fats and cholesterol in the foods you eat, and then serum cholesterol and blood lipids, which are the fats and cholesterol in your body.

Dietary fat is a highly concentrated source of calories found in the foods we eat. At 9 calories per gram, it packs more than twice the calories found in carbohydrates (starchy foods, vegetables, and fruits) or protein (lean meats and low-fat dairy products). Eating more energy than you burn off leads to weight gain. A heart-healthy diet provides 30 percent or less of its calories from fat. However, how much fat you need in your diet will depend on several factors, including your current risk for heart disease, weight, exercise patterns, and family history of disease, as well as how tightly you can control your blood glucose. You, your physician, and your dietitian will need to determine exactly how much dietary fat is right for you.

For example, if you have more than one risk factor for heart disease, such as being overweight and having a high cholesterol level, but you have good blood-glucose management, then you might benefit most from following a diet that provides 25 percent of calories from fat. However, if you have a low risk for heart disease and your blood glucose is very sensitive to carbohydrates, then you might find following a diet providing 30 to 33 percent of calories from fat more helpful for your total diabetes management. There is no magic formula here; it depends on your health and the type of lifestyle changes you can reasonably make and maintain.

The fat in the foods you eat comes in three different forms: monounsaturated, polyunsaturated, and saturated. All of these forms have *exactly the same number of calories,* but they have different effects on your health.

Monounsaturated Fats
Monounsaturated fats are found in most nuts and seeds, as well as in olives, olive oil, canola oil, peanut oil, and av-

ocados. Monounsaturated fats tend to lower blood cholesterol and may have a beneficial effect on blood-glucose levels. At the Stedman Nutrition Center, we recommend that most of the fat in your diet be monounsaturated—as much as 10 to 15 percent of your total calories. A word of caution here: this does not mean that you should eat lots of olive oil and nuts. You won't do your health any favors by eating a high-fat diet, no matter what type of fat it is.

Polyunsaturated Fats

Polyunsaturated fats are found in vegetable oils such as corn, safflower, soybean, and sunflower and are liquid at room temperature. Although they tend to lower blood cholesterol, too many polyunsaturated fats in your diet may not be healthy for you, either. Remember: all things in moderation. About 8 to 10 percent of your total calories should come from polyunsaturated fats. Polyunsaturated fats include the *omega-3 fatty acids* found in cold-water and fatty fish such as mackerel, perch, cod, salmon, tuna, and sole. The fats from these oily fish may lower the risk of heart disease; in countries where people eat a lot of these fish and little of the foods high in saturated fat, the rate of heart disease is low. However, it is not a good idea to take capsules of fish oils if you have diabetes, as they have been shown to worsen blood-glucose management and sometimes cause diarrhea. If you want to capitalize on the potential health benefits of fish oils, then choose fish as your protein source in place of meat.

Saturated Fats

Saturated fats are found in animal foods, including meat, eggs, dairy foods, and butter, as well as in oils from tropical plants such as coconut and palm. Saturated fats are solid at room temperature. Hydrogenation is a chemical process that transforms liquid oils into solids and creates trans-fatty acids, which act on your body like saturated fat. Saturated fats are the biggest culprits in heart disease, since they tend to raise blood cholesterol levels. At the Stedman Center, we recommend that you get only 2 to 7 percent of your total calories from saturated fat. The average American gets nearly 14 percent of his or her total daily calories from saturated fat, which goes far in explaining our very high rates of heart disease. This is largely owing to our very high intake of meat and of fried foods, which are often cooked in hydrogenated oils or animal fat.

Remember that when it comes to calories, a fat is a fat is a fat. But when it comes to heart disease, watch out especially for saturated fat. Nutrition is a very complex field, and not all foods are what they may seem. That is why it is a good idea to read ingredient labels. That way, you will know what you are purchasing and putting into your body. It is also important to realize that no oil contains only one kind of fat; they are all mixtures of monounsaturated, polyunsaturated, and saturated fats. Even though olive oil is made up mostly of monounsaturated fat, it is not perfectly pure.

Fat Substitutes

There are new fat substitutes on the market now, including Simplesse and olestra (known commercially as Olean). These are products the food industry uses to produce low-fat foods for consumers. When used in moderation, these products can be part of a healthy diet. However, there are two cautions with these types of fat replacers: they are generally used in salad dressings, ice creams, and other foods that are low in nutritional value but still often rich in calories, and large amounts of some of these fat substitutes may cause physical discomfort. Nonabsorbable fat substitutes, such as olestra, are used in snacks such as potato chips and french fries. Not only are these foods low in nutritional value, but large quantities of nonabsorbable fat can cause abdominal cramping and diarrhea. If you choose to include these foods in your diet, use them as you would any fat: in moderation.

Dietary Cholesterol

Dietary cholesterol is now thought to be relatively less important a health risk than either total fat intake or intake of saturated fat. Recent nutrition research has shown that it is the saturated fat you eat, not necessarily the cholesterol, that primarily raises the level of fat in your blood by signaling your liver to produce more cholesterol.

Most Americans get too much dietary cholesterol by eating animal products, including meats, eggs, and whole-milk products, which contain cholesterol produced by the livers of the animals they come from. As a nation, we consume about twice the recommended amount of cholesterol.

An important thing to know about cholesterol is that it is usually found in foods that are high in saturated fat. Since saturated fat stimulates your liver to produce cholesterol, eating these foods is like putting a double whammy on your heart health. Eating a reasonable amount of total dietary fat and limiting your saturated-fat intake is prudent advice when it comes to your good health.

Cholesterol is an essential building block of your body. You need it to make hormones, the acids and bile salts important to digestion, and cell walls. It is so important that your liver churns out cholesterol because your body does not trust that your diet will provide enough of it for you to function. The result is often too much of a good thing: high cholesterol levels in your blood. Eating a diet high in total fat, saturated fat, and cholesterol will raise your risk of heart disease, primarily by raising the levels of fats in your blood. The fats in your blood are called *lipids.* Your blood lipids include total cholesterol, HDL cholesterol, LDL cholesterol, and triglycerides.

The cholesterol in your blood is similar to the cholesterol on your plate: a waxy, fatlike substance. When levels of lipids rise too high for your body to manage, they get stuck up against the walls of your blood vessels, most of which are smaller than a drinking straw. If the blood vessels feeding your heart get clogged, then you are at risk for a heart attack. If the blood vessels feeding your brain get clogged, then you are at risk for a stroke. Your physician should check your levels of total cholesterol, HDL, LDL, and triglycerides at least every two years. It is important for you to know what your blood-fat levels are and what they mean to your health.

It is recommended that you keep your blood cholesterol (measured as "serum cholesterol") levels under 200 mg/dl. Values above this level are associated with higher risks for heart attack. When your physician checks your cholesterol level, make sure to ask her or him to request a "lipid panel." That way you will get a report of all the types of cholesterol in your blood. This information will give you a much better understanding of your risk for heart disease. You will see on your blood lipid panel report that total cholesterol breaks down into two components: HDL and LDL cholesterol.

HDL Cholesterol

HDL stands for "high-density lipoprotein." HDL cholesterol is a type of fat carried in your blood which is often referred to as "good" cholesterol. It is very small and dense and easily travels through your blood vessels without clogging them. Its function is to take fat from places of storage to places of use. In general, the higher this number, the better, because HDL cholesterol helps protect you against heart disease. As you exercise and get physically fit, you should see your levels of HDL cholesterol rise. HDL cholesterol usually falls in people with poorly controlled diabetes. Although in general HDL levels tend to be higher in women than in men, research has shown that the protective effect of being female is lost in women who have diabetes. Women need to take their heart disease risks as seriously as men—and take care of themselves.

LDL Cholesterol

LDL stands for "low-density lipoprotein." It is a type of fat carried in your blood that is often called "bad" cholesterol. It is large and fluffy-looking and plays a role in clogging your arteries by getting stuck against the sides of your artery walls and oxidized into plaque and the fatty buildup of heart disease. (To see what this looks like, smear butter against the inside of a glass: the glass represents your arteries and the butter the fatty buildup.) LDL's function is to take fat to places of storage. In general, the lower your LDL cholesterol level, the better. As you begin to eat a moderate-fat diet, exercise, and get physically fit, you should see your levels of LDL cholesterol fall. LDL cholesterol does not change much with changes in glucose control.

Triglycerides

To your blood, triglycerides are like enormous cotton balls. Ninety percent of all the fat people eat is converted into triglycerides, which are associated with heart and blood-vessel problems. Luckily for most people, triglyceride levels are high only just after meals, since these fats play a major role in moving what you just ate to its destination. People with diabetes, however, are prone to high triglyceride levels regardless of whether they have just eaten or not.

Your Blood Lipids Health Goals

Your goal for heart and cardiovascular health is low levels of total and LDL cholesterol and high levels of HDL cholesterol. The normal ranges are shown below. If your levels are not where you and your physician would like them to be, you can set a six-month goal and recheck them at that time. But remember, having good blood-fat levels is not a matter of a healthy diet alone. You can boost your chances of having healthy blood lipids by exercising regularly, avoiding smoking, managing your weight, and keeping tight control of your blood glucose.

Keeping your blood lipids in these ranges can help you minimize your risks of heart disease.

Total Cholesterol	less than 200 mg/dl
HDL Cholesterol	women: more than 55 mg/dl
	men: more than 35 mg/dl
LDL Cholesterol	less than 130 mg/dl
	(less than 115 mg/dl with
	heart disease)
Triglycerides	less than 200 mg/dl
	(less than 150 mg/dl if at
	risk for heart disease)

Managing Your Weight

Have you ever looked at a height-and-weight chart and found that you were under-tall? The problem with many of these charts is that they may present unrealistic goals and absolute guidelines. Successful diabetes management is a highly individualized process: there are no "one-size-fits-all" rules. A new measure for desirable body sizes that is better than a standard height-and-weight chart is the *body mass index* (BMI). This is a number that helps to determine how your body size is related to your health risk.

A desirable range for your BMI is between 19 and 25. A BMI under 18 is generally too low to be considered a healthy weight for an adult. At a BMI this low, you may be susceptible to osteoporosis and other chronic health problems. A BMI between 25 or 30 is considered mildly to moderately overweight and carries a slightly increased risk for weight-related health problems. Anyone in this category who has diabetes is at risk for cardiovascular disease and should consider making some lifestyle changes, such as increasing exercise and losing weight. Those whose BMI is over 30 are considered obese and at significant risk for developing weight-related health problems, especially if they have diabetes. A BMI over 40 indicates severe obesity that may require medical intervention. Use the following equation to calculate your body mass index.

$$\text{body mass index} = \frac{\text{weight (pounds)}}{(\text{height in inches})^2} \times 705$$

$$\text{example:} \quad \frac{150 \text{ lb}}{65 \text{ in}^2} \times 705 = 25$$

The best way to lose weight, lower your BMI, and reduce your health risks is to make lasting lifestyle changes, such as moderating how much fat you eat and consuming an appropriate number of calories. Many people find that they can actually eat more food but consume fewer calories simply by cutting some fat from their diet.

Keeping Track of Fat Content

The simplest and most reliable way to keep track of how much fat you consume is by counting your fat grams per day. Food manufacturers must state how many fat grams per serving any packaged food contains on nutrition labels. Label reading will be discussed in Chapter Six.

How many fat grams you need depends on the total of your health risks and your diabetes management goals. In general, a heart-healthy guideline is 25 to 30 percent of calories from fats, which is a range of 50 to 80 grams a day for a physically active woman (eating 1,800 to 2,400 calories per day) or a range of 55 to 87 grams per day for a physically active man (eating 2,000 to 2,600 calories per day). Most Americans eat more than 100 grams of fat per day.

Besides trimming your fat intake, an additional benefit of keeping fat grams within this range is that this limit almost always forces people to eat more fiber, vitamins, and minerals—substances we all know are healthy—and less cholesterol.

The following charts show you how to estimate your daily calorie need, which determines a healthy fat-gram budget for you. They are not meant to replace a visit with your physician or dietitian/nutritionist, and you may have special medical or dietary concerns that no general-information book could address. Use these tables only as a guideline to a healthier diet, not to replace your medical and professional nutritional care. Follow these other guidelines as you develop your weight-loss plan:

- If you think you should be eating less than 1,400 calories daily, you must see a registered dietitian or licensed nutritionist to have him or her help you develop a healthy eating plan. It is likely that this level of calories is too low for you to manage your diabetes successfully and will not promote permanent weight loss.

- Set your weight-loss goals for no more than 10 to 15 pounds at a time, even if you have to lose more weight than that. Your diabetes management will very likely change with every loss of about this amount of weight, so after you lose some weight, allow your body to stabilize—and allow yourself to make sure you really can maintain the lifestyle changes that led to your weight loss. Work with your diabetes care team to assess whether your diabetes management needs have changed. You may need less medication; excessive medication could put you at risk for hypoglycemia.

- If you weigh more than 300 pounds, follow a nutrition plan providing between 2,200 and 3,000 calories per day. Following anything less than 2,200 calories per day will not meet the needs of your body and will signal your body that you are starving. Signals of starvation may cause you to overeat, strongly suppress your metabolic rate, and increase your fat-storage enzymes. Although friends, relatives, or diet books may recommend a 1,200- or 1,500-calorie-per-day diet plan, this is not healthy for a larger person. Following healthy eating guidelines and moderate caloric restriction are still the way to go, even if you weigh 300 pounds or more. If you lose weight too quickly, you will be at risk for regaining it quickly, which is not thought to be healthy for your body.

How to Determine How Many Calories and How Much Fat You Should Eat

Follow the steps below to figure out how many calories you need each day.

		Answer Here
Step #1	Write your current weight here:	pounds
Step #2	Multiply your weight by 10 (weight × 10 =)	calories in BMR

This estimates your basal metabolic rate (BMR). That is the amount of calories you burn each day just to stay alive without counting exercise or other general movement.

To keep your weight in the same range but improve health:

Step #3a	Add 500 to the number in Step #2 (weight × 10 + 500 =)	calories per day

This is the right calorie intake for you if you want to improve your body composition (lose unwanted inches and tone up your body shape), maintain your weight, or lose less than 15 pounds.

To lose between 15 and 40 pounds:

Step #3b	Use the number from Step #2 as your daily calorie needs (weight × 10 =)	calories per day

To lose more than 40 pounds:

Step #3c	Subtract 500 from the number in Step #2 (weight × 10 − 500 =)	calories per day

If you weigh 350 pounds or more:

Step #3d	Subtract 1,000 from the number in Step #2 (weight × 10 − 1,000 =)	calories per day

All of these calculations assume that you are exercising 3 to 5 times a week in your appropriate training heart range.

At the Stedman Nutrition Center, we recommend a 25-percent-fat diet (see chart below). Although this is a good general health recommendation, it may not be appropriate for everyone with diabetes. The specific amount of calories, dietary fat, carbohydrate, and protein that is right for you will depend on your health risks, blood sugar control, physical activity level, and other factors.

Daily Fat Gram Amounts for Various Calorie Requirements

After you calculate how many calories you need, use this table to determine the maximum amount of fat grams you should eat each day.

Calorie Needs	20% Calories from Fat (grams)	25% Calories from Fat (grams)	30% Calories from Fat (grams)
1,200	27	33	40
1,400	31	39	46
1,600	36	44	53
1,800	40	50	60
2,000	44	56	66
2,200	48	61	73
2,400	54	67	80
2,600	58	72	86
2,800	62	77	93
3,000	66	83	100

In general, the Stedman Nutrition Center recommends a 25-percent-fat diet to help lower risks for heart disease, obesity, and certain cancers. Work with your physician and registered dietitian to determine what percentage of dietary fat is right for you.

If You Need to Lose Weight

The key to successful weight loss is a slow, steady loss through a balanced diet that continues to provide you with the nutrients you need. The Stedman Center recommends a weekly loss of no greater than between one-half and two pounds.

Many people try to lose weight by totally avoiding fat or by severely restricting their calorie intake. Some people skip meals and snacks to cut calories, while others follow a liquid diet or a very low calorie diet plan designed for quick weight loss. These short-term approaches rarely result in long-term success, and some can even endanger your health. Instead of following a starvation diet that is not likely to improve your health and may jeopardize your diabetes management, try making the lifestyle changes discussed in this book (healthy food choices, moderate exercise, stress management, and avoiding smoking). Remember, the research has shown that following a sensible diet of healthy food choices without dieting has a strong positive impact on diabetes control.

Your nutrition plan should be low enough in calories so that you will lose weight, but not so low that you feel as if you are starving or become at risk for hypoglycemia. A diet too low in calories can leave you feeling lightheaded, dizzy, weak, confused, or shaky. Always check your blood glucose if you are experiencing symptoms of hypoglycemia. Eating a sensible, healthy diet will assist you in losing weight. You can achieve this by following the Food Guide Pyramid to consume a moderate amount of a wide variety of foods.

One common problem people face when it comes to eating a healthy diet is that much of the eating we do is automatic. Research has shown that dieters underestimate the amount of food they eat and overestimate the amount they exercise. Have you ever eaten lunch at your desk, at work, in your car, or in front of the television without really thinking about it? Maybe you have sampled free foods in the grocery store or tasted a dish you're cooking without counting the calories. It can be very easy to snatch a piece of candy or a cookie from a jar and forget to count it.

One method many people have found helpful in learning to be more aware of their eating habits is to keep a food journal or record. Every food you eat affects your weight and blood-glucose and blood-fat levels. A food record can help you focus on calories you may not have realized you were consuming. You may not need to keep a food record for long, but it is a good tool to help you keep track of your eating habits and nutrition.

Ten Tips for Losing Weight

Here are ten tips to help you reach your weight goal and manage your diabetes more effectively:

1. Follow a balanced diet with only a moderate caloric restriction, not a low-calorie diet. Low-calorie diets may put you at risk for hypoglycemia and for regaining the weight you lost when you stop the diet.
2. Make gradual lifestyle changes in fitness and nutrition. Dramatic changes are difficult to keep up, leading to diet failure and often the regaining of lost weight. Making small adjustments over time will help you to make these changes permanent improvements in your lifestyle—and in your health.
3. Eat a diet moderate in fat. About 30 percent or less of your total calories every day should be from fat if you need to lose weight or have many risk factors for heart disease.
4. Eat two to four servings of fruits and three to five servings of vegetables every day. They will help you to fill up with natural vitamins, minerals, and fiber instead of fat.

5. Exercise regularly and consistently. Regular, consistent exercise is a major factor in controlling blood glucose and managing weight. Exercise burns calories, enhancing fat breakdown while toning muscle. And the effect of exercise is cumulative. If you weigh 210 pounds and walk briskly 30 minutes daily, for instance, you could lose 23 pounds through this activity alone in a year.
6. Keep track of what you are eating so that you will be made aware of any automatic food behaviors.
7. Don't skip meals or snacks. Skipping meals or snacks can cause hypoglycemia and endanger your health.
8. Eat meals and snacks at regular times.
9. Take medications at regular times.
10. Be patient. Losing weight can be very frustrating. You may have struggled with controlling your weight in the past, but remember that this new way of eating is not a fad: it is a lifelong way of keeping yourself healthy. You will have good days and not-so-good days. Don't get discouraged. Make positive changes one day at a time that will lead to improved health, weight loss, and feeling better.

The best formula for managing your weight is to exercise regularly, take your medications as prescribed, and follow your meal plan. Chapter Five will show you how to create an effective meal plan.

Meal Planning

A meal plan is the cornerstone of effective diabetes management. It's an important tool for helping you achieve the goal of balancing food, exercise, and any necessary diabetes medication. Whereas this book can help you understand your diabetes and show you *how* to eat healthfully, a personal nutrition plan is a highly individualized prescription. Your dietitian can help you create a meal plan that matches the calories, carbohydrates, protein, and fat you eat with your exercise level and the insulin in your body.

When you have your meal plan, it is crucial to be consistent regarding when you eat, how much you eat, and what types of food you eat to keep your blood-glucose levels under control. Following your meal plan will make it easier for you to give your body enough carbohydrates without overdoing it on the proteins and fats. The goal is that your food intake and your insulin will work together at the appropriate times. This balance is the key to good blood-glucose control.

Meal plans are designed so that the greatest amount

of food you will eat will be carbohydrates such as starchy grains, starchy vegetables, pasta, beans, fruits, and green leafy vegetables. Twenty years ago, scientists thought that these foods would raise blood glucose uncontrollably, but today we know that diets high in carbohydrates actually help people control their blood glucose. Diets high in complex carbohydrates, fruits, and vegetables also have been shown to help protect people against obesity, some types of cancer, and heart disease.

This chapter will explain food "exchanges" and how they can help you keep your diet in balance. In addition to keeping track of exchanges, we recommend that you count your daily grams of fat, as explained in Chapter Four. You may have learned elsewhere about counting fat exchanges, which is also an option. However, the rate at which new low-fat foods are being introduced into our supermarkets makes counting fat grams a valuable skill. Many engineered low-fat foods don't match the traditional "fat exchanges" anymore, making counting actual fat grams important. Regardless of how you wish to keep track of your dietary fat, it is very important to keep the total fat in your diet balanced, since diabetes is a risk factor for heart disease and other complications.

Your meal plan is unique to you. It depends upon more than just the status of your diabetes. Your tastes, schedule, budget, and family concerns will also affect your meal plan. Your dietitian can help you devise a meal plan that is right for you. The two of you should keep these factors in mind as you develop a meal plan:

- Nutritional needs. If you need to lose weight, your meal plan will need to be lower in fat. Follow the Food Guide Pyramid to get enough fruits and vegetables for a healthy, balanced diet.
- Schedule. If you work full time outside the home, you probably do not want to plan meals that re-

quire a lot of preparation. You may want to cook some meals ahead and freeze them so you can quickly and conveniently eat a healthy meal even after a long day at work.

- Budget. Choose foods you can afford. If you are on a limited budget, you may find it more affordable to get your protein from beans or lentils than from fish.

- Personal taste. Your dietitian may suggest fish, but if you can't stand it, don't plan a week of meals around it. Eat foods you enjoy. On the other hand, don't get locked into old food habits. If, like most Americans, you eat many highly salted or sugary foods, make gradual changes to less salty or sugary foods. Or you can try a two-week taste-bud vacation and go "cold turkey" from those high-sugar, high-salt foods. Your taste buds will adjust more quickly than you might think to the true flavors of foods. Try experimenting with a new food or dish about once a week.

Exchange Lists

Many people find that using a meal plan helps them manage their blood glucose more tightly. Meal plans are made up of a certain number of servings of foods at each meal (breakfast, lunch, dinner, and snacks). These servings are broken down into units called *exchanges*. These are based on the fact that many foods are very alike in terms of their carbohydrate, protein, fat, and calorie content and can be exchanged one for another without really changing your overall diet. It is a simple way to handle meal planning.

There are six exchange lists (which look very similar to the foods groups): Milk and Dairy Products; Starches, Grains, and Starchy Vegetables; Green, Leafy Vegetables and Other Vegetables; Fruits; Meats and Other Proteins; and Fats. Each of these kinds of foods has a different effect on your blood glucose. Below is a chart that shows how much carbohydrate, protein, fat, and calories are in one exchange of each of these kinds of foods.

Exchange List	Carbohydrate (grams)	Protein (grams)	Fat (grams)	Calories
Milk and Dairy Products				
Skim	12	8	0	90
1% low-fat	12	8	3	100
2% low-fat	12	8	5	120
Whole	12	8	8	150
Starches, Grains, and Starchy Vegetables	15	3	trace	80
Green, Leafy Vegetables and Other Vegetables	5	2	0	25
Fruits	15	0	0	60
Meats and Other Proteins				
Very lean	0	7	0–1	35
Lean	0	7	3	55
Medium-fat	0	7	5–7	75
High-fat	0	7	8–10	100
Fats	0	0	5	45

The sections that follow list the foods that fall into each of these categories. These are the *exchange lists*. They have been adapted from the lists developed by the American Diabetes Association and the American Dietetic Association. You can simply choose the number of portions specified in your meal plan from the list. You may notice that the amount of food in a serving differs slightly from food to food. The portion sizes are listed so that the nutritional content is approximately equal for each choice. Ask your dietitian for help if a food you typically eat—or particularly love—is not listed in one of these groups, or if you often eat combination foods (made from recipes that contain many ingredients) that are not listed. Almost any food can at least occasionally be worked into a meal plan for managing diabetes.

Milk and Dairy Products List

One exchange of fluid milk or plain breakfast-style yogurt gives your body about 12 grams of carbohydrate and 8 grams of protein. Milk varies widely in fat content depending on which type you choose. The amount of fat in milk is measured by percentage of butterfat. "Skim," or "nonfat," milk contains less than ½ percent butterfat, whole milk is 3.5 percent butterfat, and "low-fat" milk is 1 percent or 2 percent butterfat. Although these may sound as though they are very low in fat, the percentage does not refer to the percent of calories from fat. Whole milk is actually very high in fat (8 grams per cup) and saturated fat (5 of the 8 grams), and contains some cholesterol (34 milligrams per cup).

The Milk and Dairy Products List is divided into three parts, based on the amount of fat and number of calories: skim and very-low-fat milk, low-fat milk, and whole milk (see chart on page 54).

Milk and dairy products are probably best known nutritionally for their value in providing dietary calcium, a mineral essential for the growth, hardening, and repair of bones. Milk contains about 300 milligrams of calcium, and yogurt between 300 and 400 per exchange. In the American diet, milk on cereal provides about 60 percent of all the calcium Americans get every day. Having cereal with milk is a nutritionally sound breakfast choice. If you cannot tolerate milk or do not like it, make sure you check with your dietitian about other ways to get enough calcium in your diet.

When you look at this list you might notice something missing: cheese and frozen yogurt. Many people are surprised to learn that these do not belong to the Milk and Dairy Products group. The processing they undergo changes them to such an extent that nutritionally they no longer resemble the milk they were made from. Cheese is listed in the "Meats and Other Proteins" group, and frozen yogurt is found in "Starches, Grains, and Starchy Vegetables." There are also many foods made with milk, such as puddings, that do not fit into the milk group either. Look for them under "Combination Foods."

Skim and Very-Low-Fat Milk	
Skim milk	1 cup
½% milk	1 cup
1% milk	1 cup
Low-fat buttermilk	1 cup
Evaporated skim milk	½ cup
Dry nonfat milk	½ cup
Plain nonfat yogurt*	1 cup
Nonfat yogurt sweetened with aspartame	1 cup
Low-Fat Milk	
2% milk	1 cup
Plain low-fat yogurt (with added nonfat milk solids)*	1 cup
1% yogurt sweetened with aspartame	1 cup
Whole Milk†	
Whole milk	1 cup
Evaporated whole milk	½ cup
Whole plain yogurt*	1 cup

*Flavored yogurt has sugar and often fruit added to it. You may be able to use a fruit exchange plus a milk exchange to cover a fruit-flavored yogurt or plain yogurt to which you have added your own fresh fruit. You can also look for flavored yogurts that have been sweetened with aspartame or other non-nutritive sweeteners.

†Since whole milk is so high in fat, saturated fat, and cholesterol, it is wise to limit it in your diet. It is not recommended that adults drink whole milk, although it may be beneficial for growing children. If you have a child with diabetes, make sure you talk with your diabetes care team and your dietitian about whether or not to include whole milk in his or her meal plan.

Starches, Grains, and Starchy Vegetables

Foods from this list should make up the bulk of your diet. One serving of a food from the Starches, Grains, and Starchy Vegetables group will give your body about 15 grams of carbohydrate, 3 grams of protein, a trace of fat, and 80 calories. Some of these foods are good choices for fiber as well. For example, whole-grain breads have about 2 grams of fiber in an exchange, whereas white breads have only 1. Foods that have 3 or more grams of fiber per exchange have been asterisked. Try to include these in your diet.

Vegetables such as corn and peas are on this starch list rather than the vegetable list because their carbohydrate content makes them nutritionally more like a starch. In fact, starchy vegetables have three times the carbohydrate per serving of their green, leafy counterparts. Beans are also found on this list because of the amount of starch they contain. The USDA's new Food Guide Pyramid counts beans as proteins. For the management of diabetes, however, beans and lentils are counted as starches unless you are following a vegetarian diet. (If so, work with your dietitian to develop a meal plan that works for you.) Some canned beans are very high in sodium. Rinsing canned beans for two to three minutes under cold running water will remove half or more of the sodium.

Have foods from this category at each meal, and at snacktimes, too. When you choose starches, grains, and starchy vegetables, you can choose from any of the items on this list. You will notice that, in general, one exchange equals approximately ½ cup of cereal, grain, or pasta or 1 ounce of a bread product.

You may be surprised to learn that frozen yogurts often fit onto this list, since many of them contain 16 grams of carbohydrate, 3 grams of protein, and varying amounts of fat per ½-cup serving. But remember that it has all the sugar—and fewer of the nutrients—of fruit. Read the nutrition label to see how this fits into your meal plan. It is also a good idea to monitor your blood glucose so that you know how your body reacts to this food. Keep frozen yogurt as an occasional item only.

Cereals, Grains, and Pasta	
Cereals:	
*Bran cereals, concentrated (such as Bran Buds, All-Bran)	⅓ cup
*Bran cereals, flaked	½ cup
Other ready-to-eat unsweetened cereals	¾ cup
Shredded wheat	½ cup
Puffed cereal	1½ cups
Grape-Nuts	3 Tbsp.
Cooked cereals	½ cup
Grits (cooked)	½ cup
Granola	¼ cup plus 5 grams of fat
Grains and pastas:	
Bulgur (cooked)	½ cup
Pasta (cooked)	½ cup
Rice, white or brown (cooked)	⅓ cup
Cornmeal	2½ Tbsp.
Wheat germ	3 Tbsp.
Dried Beans, Peas, and Lentils	
Beans and peas (cooked) (such as kidney, white, split, blackeye)	⅓ cup
*Lentils (cooked)	⅓ cup
*Baked beans	¼ cup
Starchy Vegetables	
*Corn (kernels)	½ cup
*Corn on cob, 6 in.	1 piece
*Lima beans	½ cup
*Peas, green (fresh, frozen, or canned)	½ cup
*Plantain	½ cup
Potato, baked	1 small or ½ medium (3 oz.)
Potato, mashed, no added fat	½ cup
*Squash, winter (acorn, butternut)	1 cup
Yam or sweet potato	⅓ cup

Bread

Bagel	½ (1 oz.)
Bread sticks, crisp, 4 × ½ in.	2 (⅔ oz.)
Croutons, low-fat	1 cup
English muffin	½
Frankfurter or hamburger bun	½ (1 oz.)
Pita, 6 in., white or wheat	½
Plain roll, small	1 (1 oz.)
Raisin (unfrosted)	1 slice (1 oz.)
Rye or pumpernickel	1 slice (1 oz.)
Tortilla, 6 in., corn or flour	1
White (including French, Italian)	1 slice (1 oz.)
Whole wheat	1 slice (1 oz.)

Crackers and Snacks

Animal crackers	8
Graham crackers, 2½ in. square	3
Matzoh	¾ oz.
Melba toast	5 slices
Oyster crackers	24
Popcorn (popped, no fat added)	3 cups
Pretzels	¾ oz.
Ry-Krisp, 2 × 3½ in.	4
Saltine-type crackers	6
*Whole wheat crackers (no fat added)	2–4 (¾ oz.)

Starchy Foods Prepared with Fat

These foods contain about 5 grams or more of fat per exchange. Count these as 1 starch exchange plus 5 fat grams, or obtain a more accurate fat-gram content from the nutritional labeling.

Biscuit, 2½ in.	1
Chow mein noodles	½ cup
Corn bread, 2-in. cube	1 (2 oz.)
Crackers, round butter type	6
French-fried potatoes 2–3½ in.	10 (1½ oz.)
Muffin, plain, small	1
Pancakes, 4 in.	2
Stuffing, bread (prepared)	¼ cup
Taco shells, 6 in.	2
Waffle, 4½-in. square	1
Whole wheat crackers (fat added)	4–6 (1 oz.)

Other Carbohydrate Items

When using these exchange lists it is important to remember that there are no good foods or bad foods. However, there are foods for general use and those for occasional enjoyment, like cakes, cookies, and chips. Be careful to measure portions with these foods since many of them are concentrated sources of carbohydrates and often contain added fat. All of the following are one exchange.

	1 Starch Serving	Added Fat (grams)
Angel food cake	¹⁄₂₄th cake, or 1½ in. square	0
Cake, no icing	¹⁄₂₄th cake, or 1½ in. square	5
Pie, 2 crusts, fruit	¹⁄₁₈th pie	2½
Ice cream, regular	½ cup	10
Ice cream, fat-free, no added sugar	½ cup	0
Frozen yogurt, low-fat, no added sugar	½ cup	0–1
Frozen yogurt, low-fat, fat-free	⅓ cup	0–1
Brownie, small, unfrosted	2 in. square	5
Cookies	2 small	5
Vanilla wafers	5	5
Granola bar	1 bar	5
Pudding, regular, made with low-fat milk	¼ cup	0
Pudding, sugar-free, made with low-fat milk	½ cup	0
Hummus	⅓ cup	5
Potato chips	12–18 (1 oz.)	10
Tortilla chips	6–12 (1 oz.)	10

Green Leafy Vegetables and Other Vegetables

Not all vegetables are created equal. That is why some of them appear on the Starches list and some are here on the Green Leafy Vegetables and Other Vegetables List. These non-starchy vegetables are all very similar in that one exchange will give your body about 5 grams of carbohydrate, 2 grams of protein, and 25 calories. Many of these vegetables also contain 2 to 3 grams of dietary fiber, which is important for good health. You probably already know that green leafy and other vegetables are a good source of many vitamins and minerals, including folic acid. Some are even fair or good sources of calcium and iron.

Fresh and frozen vegetables tend to retain their nutrients better than canned ones, and they have less added salt. The asterisk indicates 400 milligrams or more of sodium per exchange. Rinsing canned vegetables for two to three minutes under cold running water will remove half or more of the sodium.

Unless otherwise noted, one exchange of green leafy or other vegetables is ½ cup of cooked vegetables or vegetable juice,* or 1 cup of raw vegetables.

- Artichoke (½ medium)
- Asparagus
- Beans (green, waxed, Italian)
- Bean sprouts
- Beets
- Broccoli
- Brussels sprouts
- Cabbage (cooked)
- Carrots
- Cauliflower
- Crookneck squash
- Eggplant
- Greens (collard, mustard, turnip)
- Kohlrabi
- Leeks
- Mushrooms
- Okra
- Onions
- Pea pods
- Peppers
- Rutabagas
- *Sauerkraut
- Spinach
- Tomato (one large)
- Tomato and other vegetable juices
- Turnips
- Water chestnuts
- Zucchini

Fruits

Fruit is an important part of a healthy diet, since it contains many vitamins and minerals. Each exchange of fruit contains about 15 grams of carbohydrate, 60 calories, and a trace or less of protein or fat. The exchange portion sizes listed here are based on the usual serving sizes of the most commonly eaten fruits, although not all fruits fit perfectly onto the list. (For example, one banana is usually two exchanges.) When you eat fruit, try to choose whole, unprocessed fruit as much as possible. If you are going to purchase a canned fruit, then choose the ones that are labeled "juice pack," "in its own juice," or "no added sugar."

Try to eat fruit for dessert or as a snack rather than a less nutritious sugary food. This can be particularly important if you are trying to lose weight.

Fruit can be a good source of fiber. In general, fresh, frozen, and dried fruits have about 2 grams of fiber per exchange, but we have asterisked those fruits that have 3 or more grams of fiber per exchange. Fruit juices contain very little dietary fiber. Fruit juice is also relatively high in calories and may act in your body much the same as an equal amount of soda pop, since fruit juice is made up of simple sugars. It can be easy to drink a large number of calories as fruit juice without being aware of it. If you prefer fruit juice to whole fruits, check with your dietitian about how best to work juices into your meal plan without overdoing it.

In general, one exchange of a fruit is ½ cup of fresh fruit or fruit juice, or ¼ cup of dried fruit. All fruits are raw unless otherwise noted.

Fresh, Frozen, and Unsweetened Canned Fruit	
Apple (2 in.)	1
Applesauce (unsweetened)	½ cup
Apricots (medium)	4 (5½ oz.)
Apricots, canned	½ cup
Banana (9 in.)	½
*Blackberries	¾ cup
*Blueberries	¾ cup
Cantaloupe, whole (5 in.)	⅓ (11 oz.) or 1 cup cubes
Cataloupe, cubes	1 cup
Cherries (large)	12
Cherries, canned	½ cup
Figs (2 in.)	2
Fruit cocktail, canned	½ cup
Grapefruit, whole (medium)	½
Grapefruit, segments	¾ cup
Grapes (small)	15
Honeydew, whole (medium)	1 slice (10 oz.) or 1 cup cubes
Honeydew, cubes	1 cup
Kiwi (large)	1
Mandarin orange, segments	¾ cup
Mango (small)	½
*Nectarine (2½ in.)	1
Orange (2½ in.)	1
Papaya	1 cup
Peach (2¾ in.)	1
Peaches, canned	½ cup or two halves
Pear	½ large or 1 small
Pears, canned	½ cup or 2 halves
Persimmons (medium, native)	2
Pineapple, cubes	¾ cup
Pineapple, canned	⅓ cup
Plum (2 in.)	2
*Pomegranate	½
*Raspberries	1 cup
*Strawberries (whole)	1¼ cups
*Tangerine (2½ in.)	2
Watermelon, cubes	1¼ cups

Dried Fruit	
*Apples	4 rings
*Apricots	8 halves
Dates	2½ medium
*Figs	1½
*Prunes	3 medium
Raisins	2 Tbsp.
Fruit Juice	
Apple juice and cider	½ cup
Cranberry juice cocktail	⅓ cup
Grapefruit juice	½ cup
Grape juice	⅓ cup
Orange juice	½ cup
Pineapple juice	½ cup
Prune juice	⅓ cup

Meats and Other Proteins

Current health guidelines call for moderation in the consumption of meats and other proteins. Your body can manage healthfully with as few as 6 exchanges (about 6 ounces) of meat per day, since that will meet all of your body's health needs. Limiting your intake of meats and other proteins can help you lower your risks for heart and blood-vessel disease, since many of these foods are high in fat, saturated fat, and cholesterol. Try to select proteins that are very lean, lean, or medium-fat when you include them at your meals. Limit choices from the high-fat list to no more than three times per week or less, and be particularly careful when ordering meat at restaurants. Restaurants generally serve the higher-fat cuts of meat.

Here are some tips to help you cook healthfully with meats and other proteins:

- Choose the leanest meats and other proteins as often as possible.

- Always trim all visible fat from meat before and after cooking, and remove the skin.
- Grill, broil, bake, roast, or boil meats and other proteins rather than frying them in oil or other added fat. Nonstick cooking sprays and nonstick pans are essential to the healthful cooking of meats and other proteins.
- If you are coating a meat such as chicken, dip it first in nonfat yogurt or egg white and then in flour, crushed corn flakes, or fresh bread crumbs. (See the recipe section for some ideas about cooking batter-coated foods.)
- Remember that until you are well skilled at judging portions by sight, it is a good idea to weigh them to make sure you aren't eating too much meat or other proteins. Four ounces of raw meat yield about 3 ounces cooked, which looks about the same as a deck of cards.

In general, one exchange equals approximately 1 ounce, though some foods do differ. Here is a guide to judging portions:

2 ounces of meat (two meat exchanges) equals
    1 small chicken leg or thigh
    ½ cup cottage cheese or tuna
3 ounces of meat (three meat exchanges) equals
    1 medium pork chop
    1 small hamburger
    ½ of a whole chicken breast
    1 fish fillet (unbreaded)
    Cooked meat about the size of a deck of cards

One exchange of meats or other protein will give your body about 7 grams of protein and no carbohydrates, as the chart below shows. The amount of fat and calories will depend on the type of meat or other protein you choose. Meats and Other Proteins are usually divided into four categories: very lean, lean, medium-fat, and high-fat. Note that cheese falls into the Meats and Other Proteins category and not into the Milk and Dairy Products group.

Some meat choices are also very high in sodium. We have asterisked those that are higher than 400 milligrams per exchange. Very lean meats are now more readily available. The nutritional labeling on the package will indicate if your meat or other protein choice fits into this category.

Very Lean Meats and Other Proteins	
Poultry:	
White meat chicken, turkey, Cornish hen without skin	1 oz.
Fish:	
Fresh or frozen cod, flounder, haddock, halibut, trout, fresh tuna, tuna canned in water	1 oz.
Shellfish:	
Clams, crab, lobster, scallops, shrimp, imitation shellfish	1 oz.
Game:	
Wild duck or pheasant without skin, venison, buffalo, ostrich	1 oz.
Cheese:	
Nonfat or low-fat cottage cheese	¼ cup
Fat-free cheese	1 oz.
Any cheese product with 1 gram or less fat per ounce	1 oz.
Other:	
Processed sandwich meats with 1 gram or less fat per ounce (deli thin, shaved meats, chipped beef,* turkey ham)	1 oz.
Egg whites	2
Egg substitutes	¼ cup
Hot dogs* or imitation hot dogs* with 1 gram or less fat per ounce	1 oz.

| †Kidney | 1 oz. |
| Sausage with 1 gram or less fat per ounce | 1 oz. |

Count as one very lean meat and one starch choice:

| Dried Beans, peas, lentils (cooked) | ½ cup |

†*This is high in cholesterol.*

Lean Meats and Other Proteins

Beef:

| USDA Select or Choice grades of lean beef, such as round, sirloin, and flank steak; tenderloin; and chipped beef,* rib, chuck, or rump roast; T-bone, Porterhouse, or cubed steak; ground round | 1 oz. |

Pork:

| Lean pork, such as fresh ham; canned, cured, or boiled ham;* Canadian bacon;* tenderloin | 1 oz. |

Lamb:

| Roast, chop, leg | 1 oz. |

Veal:

| Lean chop, roast | 1 oz. |

Poultry:

Dark meat chicken, turkey, Cornish hen without skin	1 oz.
White meat chicken with skin	1 oz.
Domestic duck or goose without skin, fat drained	1 oz.

Fish:

Salmon, catfish	1 oz.
Oysters	6 medium
Tuna canned in oil (drained)	2 oz.
Herring, smoked or pickled (no cream)	1 oz.
Sardines canned in oil, drained	2 medium

Game:

Rabbit, squirrel	1 oz.
Wild goose without skin	1 oz.
Quail without skin	1 oz.

Cheese:

4.5%-fat cottage cheese	2 oz.
Grated Parmesan	2 Tbsp.
Dried cheeses* (with 55 calories or less per ounce)	1 oz.
Mysost	1 oz.

Lean Meats and Other Proteins *(cont'd.)*

Other:

Hot dogs or 95%-fat-free lunch meats* or lunch meats with 3 grams or less fat per ounce	1½ oz.

Medium-Fat Meats and Other Proteins

Beef:

Most beef products fall into this category, including all ground beef, short ribs, corned beef, prime meats well trimmed of fat, and meat loaf (count sauce separately)	1 oz.

Pork:

Most pork products fall into this category, including chops, loin roast, Boston butt, and cutlets	1 oz.

Lamb:

Rib roast, ground	1 oz.

Veal:

Cutlet (ground or cubed, unbreaded)	1 oz.

Poultry:

Dark meat chicken with skin, ground turkey, ground chicken, fried chicken with skin	1 oz.

Fish:

Any fried fish	2 oz.

Cheese:

Skim or part-skim milk cheeses including

Ricotta	2 oz.
Mozzarella	2 oz.
Diet cheeses	1 oz.
Feta cheese*	1 oz.
Neufchâtel	1 oz.
Camembert	1 oz.

Other:

86%-fat-free lunch meats	1 oz.
†Egg	1
Egg substitutes with 56–80 calories per ¼ cup	2 oz.
Tofu (2½ × 2¾ × 1 in.)	4 oz.
Tempeh	2 oz.
Soy milk	8 oz.

†*Eggs are high in cholesterol and should be limited to 3 per week.*

High-Fat Meats and Other Proteins

These items are high in saturated fats, cholesterol, and calories. Choose them fewer than three times per week if you choose them at all.

Pork:

Spareribs, ground pork, pork sausage (patty or link)*	1 oz.

Cheese:

All whole-milk cheeses such as American,* blue,*
  Cheddar, Monterey Jack, Swiss, Colby, brick,
  Muenster, and provolone, and specialty cheeses
  such as Brie, caraway, Cheshire, Edam, fontina,
  Gouda, Gjetost, Gruyère, Limburger, Romano, hard
  Parmesan, and Tilsit   1 oz.

Other:

Lunch meats* such as bologna, salami, and pimento loaf with 8 grams or more fat per ounce	1 oz.
Sausage* such as Polish and Italian smoked	1 oz.
Knockwurst*	1 oz.
Bratwurst	1 oz.
Turkey or chicken frankfurter*	1
Peanut butter	1 Tbsp.

Count as one high-fat meat plus count the fat grams:

Beef, pork, or combination frankfurter*	1

Fat

We recommend that you count your fat grams to keep track of them rather than counting fat exchanges. There are so many new products and foods available today that don't fit the traditional exchanges when it comes to fat. However, you can count fat exchanges if you prefer. Mostly the foods on this list are all fat, although some may have small amounts of protein as well. Remember to measure fats carefully, because small errors in portion sizes add up very quickly to a lot of fat and calories.

It is prudent advice for everyone to limit saturated fats and to use unsaturated fats instead. But remember to keep your total diet moderate in fat. People often make the mistake of adding monounsaturated fats like olive oil to their diet rather than cutting back on total fat and switching to less-saturated fats.

Since there is wide variation in sodium content in the foods available today, make sure you read the nutrition labeling for information about sodium if that is a health issue for you. Fats that contain 300 or more milligrams of sodium per exchange are asterisked.

These lists are divided by type of fat: unsaturated (containing monounsaturated and polyunsaturated) and saturated. Each exchange contains about 5 grams of fat and 45 calories.

Unsaturated Fats	
Margarine, vegetable oil, mayonnaise	1 tsp.
Diet margarine, diet mayonnaise	1 Tbsp.
Salad dressing	1 Tbsp.
Diet salad dressing	2 Tbsp.
Olives	10 small or 8 large
Avocado	⅛ medium
Nuts and seeds (½ ounce contains between 4 and 9 grams of fat):	
Almonds (dry roasted)	6 whole
Cashews (dry roasted), sunflower seeds, or pine nuts	1 Tbsp.
Pecans	2
Peanuts	18 small
Hazelnuts	4
Pumpkin seeds	1 oz.
(One tablespoon of fat-free salad dressing is a free food.)	

Saturated Fats	
Butter	1 tsp.
Bacon	1 slice
Coconut (shredded)	2 Tbsp.
Coffee whitener, liquid	2 Tbsp.
Coffee whitener, powder	2 tsp.
Light cream	2 Tbsp.
Sour cream	2 Tbsp.

Heavy (whipping) cream	1 Tbsp.
Cream, half-and-half	2 Tbsp.
Cream cheese, regular	1 Tbsp. (½ oz.)
Cream cheese, reduced-fat	2 Tbsp. (1 oz.)
*Salt pork, fried	1 oz.

Free Foods

There are some foods that contain less than 20 calories per serving and should not have a notable impact on your blood glucose. For items that have no specific serving size noted, it will be difficult to eat enough of them to affect your blood glucose strongly. For those items that have a specific portion size listed, you can have two or three exchanges per day as long as you spread them out through the day. Those that have 400 milligrams or more of sodium per exchange are asterisked.

Drinks	
Bouillon* or broth without fat	Coffee and tea
Bouillon, low-sodium	Drink mixes, sugar-free
Carbonated drinks, sugar-free	Tonic water, sugar-free
Carbonated water	Nonstick pan spray
Club soda	
Cocoa powder, unsweetened (1 Tbsp.)	
Vegetables	
Celery (2 stalks)	Hot peppers (2 peppers)
Green onion	
Sweet Substitutes	
Hard candy, sugar-free (1 candy)	Sugar substitutes (saccharin, aspartame, acesulfame K)
Gelatin, sugar-free	Whipped topping, regular or light (2 Tbsp.)
Gum, sugar-free	
Jam and jelly, sugar-free (2 tsp.)	
Pancake syrup, sugar-free (2 Tbsp.)	

Fat-Free or Low-Fat Foods	
Cream cheese, fat-free	1 Tbsp.
Creamers, non-dairy, liquid	1 Tbsp.
Salsa	¼ cup
Mayonnaise, reduced-fat	1 tsp.
Mayonnaise, fat-free	1 Tbsp.
Margarine, fat-free	4 Tbsp.
Margarine, reduced-fat	1 tsp.
Nonstick cooking spray	
Sour cream, fat-free or reduced-fat	1 Tbsp.

Condiments

Catsup (1 Tbsp.)	Low-calorie salad dressing
Horseradish	(2 Tbsp.)
Mustard	Taco sauce (1 Tbsp.)
Dill pickles,* unsweetened	Vinegar
(1½ large)	

Seasonings

Flavoring extracts (vanilla, almond, walnut, peppermint, butter, lemon, etc.)	Lime juice
	Onion powder
	Pimento
Garlic	Spices (mint, cinnamon,
Garlic powder	curry, dill, celery seeds,
Herbs (basil, chives, oregano, etc.), fresh or dried	chili powder, lemon pepper, pepper, paprika)
Hot-pepper sauce	Soy sauce*
Lemon	Soy sauce, low-sodium ("lite")
Lemon juice	Wine used in cooking (¼ cup)
Lime	Worcestershire sauce*

Combination Foods

Many of the foods we eat are made from recipes containing many ingredients and so do not neatly fit into an exchange list. For example, a thin-crust vegetable pizza has bread from the crust, protein from the cheese, and vegetables from the toppings, plus fat grams. An average serving of a pizza such as this would give you two starch exchanges, one protein exchange (medium-fat), and about 5 grams of fat. If there are enough vegetables on the topping, it might give you one exchange of vegetables as well. The total fat content would be about 10 grams (5 grams from the protein exchange, plus 5 grams added fat).

Below is a list of some common combination foods. If you have foods you like to eat that are not listed here, check with your dietitian about how you can work these into your meal plan. You can use the nutrition labeling on packages of prepared foods and the chart of carbohydrate, protein, and fat content on page 52 to figure out the exchange values of most combination foods.

Food	Amount	Exchanges
Potpie	1 (7 oz.)	
Cheese pizza, thin crust*	¼ of 10-in. (5-oz.) pizza	2 starch, 1 medium-fat meat, plus 5 grams of fat
Pizza, meat topping, thin crust	¼ of 10-in. (5-oz.) pizza	2 starch, 2 medium-fat meat, plus 10 grams of fat
Chili with beans*	1 cup (8 oz.)	2 starch, 2 medium-fat meat, plus 17 grams of fat
Tuna-noodle casserole,* lasagne, chili with beans, spaghetti and meatballs, macaroni and cheese	1 cup (8 oz.)	2 starch, 2 medium-fat meat
Chow mein (without noodles or rice)*	2 cups (16 oz.)	1 starch, 2 lean meat
Bean soup*†	1 cup (8 oz.)	1 starch, 1 very lean meat
Chunky soups (all varieties)*	1 can (10¾ oz.)	1 starch, 1 vegetable, 1 medium-fat meat
Cream soups (made with water)*	1 cup (8 oz.)	1 starch, 1 fat
Vegetable* or broth-type soups	1 cup (8 oz.)	1 starch
Tomato soup (made with water)	1 cup (8 oz.)	1 starch

Food	Amount	Exchanges
Split pea soup (made with water)	½ cup (4 oz.)	1 starch
Sugar-free pudding (made with skim milk)	½ cup (4 oz.)	1 starch
†If beans are used as a meat, substitute:		
Dried beans, peas, lentils	1 cup (cooked)	2 starch, 1 lean meat, plus 3 grams of fat

Eating Consistently

The key to a successful meal plan is to eat consistent meals and snacks. Eating consistently according to your meal plan will help you achieve better glucose control because your meal plan is designed to keep your blood-glucose levels normal.

It is important to recognize that people eat in different ways. Some people like three square meals a day, while others like to plan a snack or two. You need to do what is best for you. If you want a snack, incorporate it into your meal plan. The important thing is to be consistent and not to change eating times or the amount eaten. Suppose you eat breakfast at 6:30 A.M. You might get pretty hungry before lunch at 12:30 P.M. A snack between 9:00 and 10:00 A.M. might be just what the dietitian ordered to keep blood sugars from dipping too low and help prevent overeating at lunchtime.

Snacks in the evening before bedtime work for many people to help prevent low blood glucose during the night. Try to choose one that is low in fat. Many people find that a milk exchange, such as a cup of low-fat or nonfat yogurt, works to help them manage their blood glucose through the night. Others find that a small bowl of cereal with milk works well. In general, any food can be used as a snack, as long as it follows the consistency rule: same type, same time, same amount. Always take any prescribed medication with your meals or snacks, as instructed by your physician; take medications about half an hour before a meal.

Remember these tips for eating consistently:

- Eat meals and snacks at about the same time daily.
- Keep serving sizes consistent.
- Do not stray from your meal plan.

Sick Days

When you are ill, you often eat less. Yet fever and illness tend to raise blood-glucose levels. So when you are sick it is important to continue taking any insulin or diabetes pills prescribed by your doctor. It is also important to try to keep eating the same amount of carbohydrates as usual, although it may be easier to spread them out throughout the day, rather than to concentrate them in three meals. Easy-to-digest foods such as crackers and bananas may go down more easily than some other foods. It is also important to continue drinking liquids so that you do not become dehydrated. Here are some tips to remember when you are sick:

- Continue to take your pills or insulin, even if you are not eating as much as you normally do.
- Monitor your blood glucose frequently. Many people find four times a day to be most helpful: before each meal and at bedtime.
- Test your urine for ketones if your blood glucose is more than 240 mg/dl.
- If you can't tolerate regular foods, replace carbohydrates in your meal plan with liquid, semiliquid,

or soft foods. The carbohydrate source is not as important as being able to find something you can tolerate. Some examples of liquid carbohydrate sources are juice, soda, soup, gelatin, and Popsicles.

- If your blood glucose is below 240 mg/dl, consume 15 grams of carbohydrate (such as ½ cup apple juice or applesauce every one to two hours, or 50 grams of carbohydrate (such as 1 cup juice and 3/4 cup applesauce or 10 saltine crackers, 1 cup soup, and ½ cup juice) every three to four hours.
- Drink 8 to 12 ounces of fluid (water, broth, tea, etc.) each hour. A carbohydrate source can also be your fluid source.
- If you are vomiting, have diarrhea, or are running a fever, consume small amounts of salted foods and liquids more frequently to replace lost electrolytes, such as sodium and potassium.
- Call your doctor's office if you have a fever of 101.5 degrees F. or higher, vomiting persists for more than a few hours, or you are unable to keep anything in your stomach.

Children's Special Needs

Children with diabetes basically follow the same diet as adults with diabetes. Children generally need more calories than adults because they are growing. Those extra calories should not come from extremely fatty foods, as children become vulnerable to diabetes complications such as heart disease as they grow older. It is especially important that children eat a balanced diet so that they will receive all the nutrients they need to build strong bodies.

That may present a special challenge for parents. Young children can be finicky eaters, while teens tend to lead hectic lives that make eating consistently difficult. More sensitive food issues can surface among children with diabetes because of peer pressure or as they come to terms with the disease. Teens may eat too much in an attempt to fit in with their peers, and young children may rebel against regimented diets.

You can avoid or minimize these problems by talking openly with your child about his or her diabetes and letting him or her make as many decisions as possible about how to manage the disease. Children should have a say in what foods they eat. Present as many food choices as possible. Let them help plan their meals, taking into account their tastes and schedule. Teach your child about nutrition, meal plans, and exchanges in an inviting way so that he is inclined to be an active participant in his diabetes management. Create a pleasant mealtime atmosphere so that dinnertime does not become a battlefield for resolving issues that have nothing to do with food.

Remember, a diabetes diet is a healthy diet for everyone, so serve the entire family the same low-fat, nutritious meals that you desire your child to eat. The child will not feel singled out, and your family will be healthier. Stock your cupboards and refrigerator with healthy, low-fat snack choices so that children develop healthy eating habits. Praise good choices. As children get older they can test their own blood and urine, which may help give them a sense of empowerment in managing their diabetes.

Because children with diabetes cannot make insulin and require insulin injections, eating consistent meals and snacks is important to avoid hypoglycemia. Carbohydrate snacks before exercise and at bedtime can help avoid insulin reactions. You also can work with your doctor or dietitian on intensive diabetes management. This is the newest way of treating diabetes, in which multiple insulin injections are given each day. But medications are fitted to eating, rather than eating being fitted to medications. You will need to monitor your child's blood glucose more often and injections will be necessary more frequently, but this method may give you or your child more flexibility and better blood-glucose control. Although there are also insulin pumps available that can help achieve this same goal without the need for multiple injections, these intensive regimens may not be appropriate for all young children.

Your diabetes care team can help you with ideas and steer you to support services for raising a child who has diabetes.

Carbohydrate Counting

An alternative system for meal planning for people who require insulin is *carbohydrate counting*. Carbohydrate counting involves keeping track of the grams of carbohydrates, rather than the exchanges, that you eat. This method concentrates on carbohydrates found in starchy foods and sugars because they have the most impact on your blood glucose. It operates on the theory that there is a ratio between the number of grams of carbohydrate a person consumes and the amount of insulin he or she requires to use those carbohydrates. Once you figure out your insulin-to-carbohydrate ratio, you can determine how many carbohydrate choices you should eat daily to keep your blood-glucose levels at their optimal levels. People who use carbohydrate counting often use the ADA Exchange Lists to figure out their carbohydrate choices for the day. They also read food labels to find out how many carbohydrate grams are in the foods they eat.

The main advantage of this method is that you need only keep track of two kinds of food: carbohydrates for glucose control and fats for a heart-healthy diet. The disadvantages, however, may outweigh the advantages. By concentrating only on carbohydrates, people may ignore other important nutrients in foods and may be less likely to eat a balanced diet. And it is vital to keep track of fat grams regardless of what nutritional method you use to manage your diabetes, even though straight carbohydrate-counting guides may not mention the importance of fat grams.

Computing your insulin-to-carbohydrate ratio can also be complicated. If you are interested in using carbohydrate counting to control your diabetes, talk with your dietitian or diabetes educator. She or he can help you determine whether carbohydrate counting is a feasible method of diabetes control for you.

Once you've put together a meal plan, you'll want to stock your kitchen with ingredients to create nutritious and inviting meals. Chapter Six will show you how to shop for a healthy variety of foods that fit into your meal plan.

Shopping

Every food you need to create a healthy diet for diabetes management can be found in your local supermarket. You can usually make the best, and most economical, choices by planning ahead. Probably the best thing you can do to make shopping quick and easy is to work from a basic set of five to ten of your favorite and healthiest recipes. The basic ingredients for these recipes will make up your "staples" list for grocery shopping.

Following your staples list and buying only a few special items will help you control grocery shopping costs and reduce wasted food. Besides that, you will be able to throw together nutritious meals in a snap without having to plan menus a week in advance. While some people find that planning the week's meals is helpful, many people find it tedious and frustrating. By working from a basic set of recipes, you will have the flexibility to eat what you like and still follow your meal plan.

After developing your staples list, the next most important skill for healthy shopping is understanding how to read a food label. Food labels can answer your nutrition questions about the foods you are buying.

Food Labeling

In May 1994, the Food and Drug Administration introduced a new, more informative, accurate, and useful "Nutrition Facts" label for most packaged foods sold in grocery stores. These labels are designed to help clear up confusion about the nutritional value of supermarket products, help consumers choose healthier diets, and give food companies an incentive to improve the nutritional qualities of their products.

In addition to information about calories, fat, carbohydrates, sodium, protein, iron, calcium, and vitamins, you can also get information about the amount per serving of saturated fat, cholesterol, dietary fiber, and other nutrients that are of major health concern to shoppers. When you know how to read it, the "Nutrition Facts" labeling makes it easier to understand what you eat.

You will usually find the "Nutrition Facts" box on the back or side of a package. The information is presented in large type on a white or neutral background for easy reading. Look for the serving size at the top of the box. Serving sizes are designed to reflect the amount people actually eat, making it easy to compare the nutritional qualities of similar foods.

Under the serving size you will find how many calories a serving contains and how many of these calories are from fat. Beneath that is listed how many grams the food contains of fat, saturated fat, cholesterol, sodium, carbohydrates, protein, and other nutrients.

To the right is a column headed "% Daily Value." The daily values are based on a 2,000-calorie-per-day diet. The "% Daily Value" tells you at a glance whether a food is high or low in fat, cholesterol, sodium, carbohydrates, protein, and fiber in relation to federal dietary recommendations. Although 2,000 calories is the amount of energy (calories) needed by the average woman, you might need slightly more or less depending on your age, sex, height, weight, and activity level.

In the lower portion of the box, other nutrients in the food may be listed. However, it is important to realize that they will be listed only as their "% Daily Value," not as their total amount in grams or milligrams as are the nutrients on the upper portion of the label.

When you see a food labeled "Light" or "Low-Fat" you can rest assured that those words have a standard meaning—although it may not be what you think they mean. (You may remember when a product would be labeled "Light" in reference to color or texture.)

Any health claim must be supported by scientific evidence. For instance, only foods that are low in fat, saturated fat, and cholesterol can carry the statement "While many factors affect heart disease, diets low in saturated fat and cholesterol may reduce the risk of this disease." The federal laws that mandate labeling have been designed to protect you, the consumer, from food misinformation.

It is important to realize, however, that health is a complex picture with many interrelated parts. What you eat does not solely determine your health. For example, eating a healthy diet cannot make up for the risks of stroke, heart disease, and cancer caused by smoking tobacco. Although diet is an important part of your total health profile, it is still just a single part.

Health Claims

As you shop, you may notice that some food products make certain claims about their health benefits. These claims will tell you the link between certain nutrients and risk factors for specific diseases. The FDA allows eight specific health claims to be carried on some foods, since the scientific research has clearly shown the relationship between the nutrient and the prevention or treatment of a specific disease. The claims include statements about the following:

- fat and the greater risk for some types of cancer
- saturated fat and cholesterol and the greater risk for heart disease
- sodium and the greater risk for hypertension
- fruits, vegetables, and grains that contain soluble fiber and the lower risk for heart disease
- fiber-containing grain products, fruits, and vegetables and the lower risk for certain types of cancer
- fruits and vegetables and the lower risk for certain types of cancer
- folic acid and the lower risk for pregnant women of bearing children with neural-tube defects
- calcium-rich foods and the lower risk for osteoporosis

Consumers may find other claims about nutrient content on food labels. Often, they appear on the front so that shoppers can readily see them. These claims signal that the food contains desirable levels of certain nutrients. The following table explains the approved claims and what they mean.

Key Words on the New Food Label	
Key Words	**What They Mean**
Fat	
Fat free	less than 0.5 gram of fat per serving
Low fat	3 grams or less of fat per serving

Key Words	What They Mean
Reduced or less fat	at least 25% less fat per serving than the food to which it is being compared

Saturated Fat

Key Words	What They Mean
Saturated fat free	less than 0.5 gram of saturated fat and less than 0.5 gram of trans-fatty acids per serving
Low saturated fat	1 gram or less of saturated fat per serving and 15% or less of calories from saturated fat
Reduced or less saturated fat	at least 25% less saturated fat per serving than the food to which it is being compared

Cholesterol

Key Words	What They Mean
Cholesterol free	less than 2 mg of cholesterol and 2 or fewer grams of saturated fat per serving
Low cholesterol	20 mg or less of cholesterol and 2 grams or less of saturated fat per serving, and if the serving is less than 30 grams or 2 tablespoons, per 50 grams of the food
Reduced or less cholesterol	at least 25% less cholesterol than the food to which it is being compared, and 2 or less grams of saturated fat per serving

The following claims can be used to describe meat, poultry, seafood, and game:

Key Words	What They Mean
Extra lean	less than 5 grams of fat, less than 2 grams of saturated fat, and less than 95 mg of cholesterol per serving and per 100 grams

Key Words	What They Mean
Lean	less than 10 grams of fat, less than 4.5 grams of saturated fat, and less than 95 mg of cholesterol per serving (usually 3 ounces in 100 grams)
Calories, Fat, and Sodium	
Light or lite	one-third fewer calories or half the fat of the food to which it is being compared; if the food derives 50 percent or more of its calories from fat, the reduction must be 50 percent of the fat
	or
	a "low calorie," "low fat" food whose sodium content has been reduced by 50 percent or less than the food to which it is being compared; may be used on foods that are not "low calorie" or "low fat"
Fiber	
High fiber	5 grams or more of fiber per serving
Good source of fiber	2.5 to 4.9 grams of fiber per serving
More or added fiber	2.5 grams or more of fiber per serving than the food to which it is being compared
Sugar	
Sugar free	less than 0.5 gram of sugar per serving
No added sugar	no sugar or ingredients that functionally substitute for sugar (such as fruit juice) or ingredients made with added sugar (such as jam)

Key Words on the New Food Label *(cont'd.)*	
Key Words	**What They Mean**
Reduced sugar	at least 25% less sugar than the food to which it is being compared
Health	
Healthy	a "low fat," "low saturated fat" food with 60 mg or less of cholesterol per serving
	or
	"extra lean" meat, poultry, seafood, or game with 60 mg or less of cholesterol per serving
	and
	at least 10% of Daily Value per serving for one or more of the following: vitamin A, vitamin C, iron, calcium, protein, and fiber
	and
	480 mg or less of sodium per serving and, if the serving is less than 30 grams or 2 tablespoons, per 50 grams of the food

Ingredients List

Food manufacturers must list the ingredients in a product on the food label. These ingredients are listed in order of weight, from the heaviest to the lightest. For example, the following label on a loaf of sunflower bread tells us that it contains mostly organically grown whole-wheat flour. There is less honey by weight than either sunflower seeds or canola oil.

Ingredients: organically grown whole wheat flour, water, sunflower seeds, organic whole wheat gluten, cold-pressed canola oil, honey, yeast, salt

Now let's look at another ingredients list. This one is for a fat-free chocolate chip "blondie" and is far more difficult to interpret.

Ingredients: pure cane sugar, wheat flour, water, high fructose corn syrup, rice syrup, whey protein concentrate, egg whites, raisin puree, dried plum puree, date puree, chocolate liquor, glycerine, molasses, nonfat dry milk, wheat fiber, natural vanilla flavor, fructose, baking soda, salt, cocoa butter.

It might be tempting to pick up this food at the grocery store because it says "fat free" on the label. But take a look at the ingredients. Three of the first five ingredients are some type of sugar. According to the nutrition label, each 1.4-ounce serving contains 120 calories, no fat, 29 grams of carbohydrate, and 2 grams of protein, so you aren't saving any calories over a standard brownie. This is true of many fat-free desserts—the manufacturers often replace the fat with sugar, and the calories stay the same.

If your blood glucose is in good control, you eat a healthy diet, and excess weight is not an issue for you, you probably could work this food into your diet as a bread/starch and a fruit exchange. But consider its nutritional value. Does a blondie give your body the nutrients that a serving of bread/starch and a fruit would? No! This is an empty-calorie food no matter how you count it. Beware of "fat free" foods (particularly desserts and snacks) in the grocery store. Despite their no-fat status, they may not do your diabetes any favors. And remember: a healthy diet is not made up of desserts and snack foods, no matter how little fat they have in them.

As a person with diabetes, it will be particularly important for you to read nutritional labels and ingredients lists so that you can make wise shopping choices that are both moderate or low in fat while high in nutrition. If any of the following is among the first few ingredients on a nutrition label, the food may be high in fat:

- Any kind of oil or fat, including
    animal fat (bacon, beef, chicken, lard)
    butter
    coconut or coconut oil
    palm or palm kernel oil
    vegetable oil (sunflower, safflower, peanut, olive)
- cream or cream sauce (unless made with acceptable ingredients)
- whole egg and egg yolk solids
- hydrogenated oil
- chocolate or cocoa butter
- whole milk solids
- vegetable shortening
- cheese (those made with part skim milk are acceptable for occasional use)

You may also want to check the ingredients label for the amount of sodium in prepared foods. The Stedman Center recommends that most people limit their sodium intake to between 1,100 and 3,300 milligrams daily. If you have high blood pressure, consider limiting it to 2,200 milligrams a day. Sodium is found in common table salt, as well as in monosodium glutamate (MSG) and sodium additives such as sodium benzoate, sodium nitrate, sodium bicarbonate, and sodium phosphate.

Shop the Perimeter

Remember the Food Guide Pyramid we discussed in Chapter Three? In general, the perimeter of the grocery store is like a trip through the pyramid. Most of the foods from each category are grouped together. That's where you'll find fresh foods such as fruits, vegetables, milk, and fish. Shopping the perimeter is a sensible route for health-conscious consumers who want to stock up on nutritious foods before they venture into the interior aisles, which tend to be filled with packaged foods that contain more sugar, fat, and salt.

Produce Section

Start shopping in the produce section—usually the first section shoppers encounter after walking through the front door. Fill your cart with fresh vegetables and fruits. These are low in fat and high in vitamins and fiber, and should make up a major portion of your diet. The National Cancer Institute's "5-a-Day" campaign calls for eating at least five servings of fruits and vegetables daily to help lower your risks for cancer (although your specific meal plan may call for more than five servings).

As you make changes in your diet, try to include fruits for desserts and snacks. You might find that you don't miss the heavier desserts and can be easily satisfied with fresh fruit or a fruit-based treat. Check out the recipes in Chapter Seven for some delicious suggestions.

If you have questions about a specific fruit or vegetable, look for the nutritional facts now posted in most grocery stores. These posters and signs will tell you what the best-selling fruits and vegetables are giving your body in terms of nutrition.

Meat and Fish Counter

At the meat counter you will find foods high in protein—and also saturated fat. Most supermarket meat cuts are

"Choice" grade, but there is a leaner cut called "Select." Read the packaging to choose the leanest cuts of beef, and trim them of visible fat before cooking. When buying ground beef, ask the butcher to grind one of the leanest cuts—eye of round, round tip, top round, top loin, tenderloin, or sirloin—or buy extra-lean ground beef that is 9 percent fat or less. The recommended limit for beef is one or two 3-ounce servings weekly.

The meat counter offers several satisfying and healthier alternatives to beef. Buy the new low-fat hot dogs (but be careful, as many are high in sodium). Select chicken or more exotic alternatives such as Cornish hen, which are low in fat as long as you cook them without skin.

You will also find a variety of fish. The Stedman Center recommends that you include fish as part of a healthy diet two or three times a week. Buy fish high in omega-3 fatty acids, which may help to raise your levels of HDL—the "good" cholesterol—and lower your risk for heart disease. These fish include cod, herring, mackerel, perch, salmon, sole, and tuna.

Bakery Section

The bakery counter is an important stop because grains form the base of the Food Guide Pyramid and should make up the bulk of your diet. However, it is important to read the labels on baked goods and to remember that while bread is usually low in fat, most bakery sweets are high in total fat and saturated fat. Many commercial bakery products are prepared with saturated fat such as lard, partially hydrogenated vegetable oil, coconut oil, or palm oil.

Also look carefully at muffins before you buy them. Many muffins are higher in fat than a doughnut. It is not unusual for a fist-sized muffin to contain 25 or 30 grams of fat. Croissants are similar to high-fat muffins, since they derive half of their calories from fat. If there is no nutritional labeling on the product, we recommend that you do not buy it.

Choose baked goods that are made from whole grains, as they will be higher in fiber. Look for bread that lists 100 percent whole wheat as the first ingredient, since it contains nearly twice the amount of fiber and more vitamins and minerals than white bread. The following products tend to be low in fat: bread, bagels, pasta, flour tortillas (made without lard), corn tortillas, and pita bread.

Dairy Section

The dairy section is full of foods rich in calcium and protein, but also high in saturated fat. Choose nonfat dairy products such as skim milk. "Low-fat" milk is not really so low in fat, because the term refers to the amount of fat by weight, as the following chart illustrates:

Type of Milk	Calories	Fat (in grams)	% Calories from Fat
Skim	90	0	0
½%	90	1	10
1%	110	2	16
2%	120	5	37
Whole	150	8	48

Choose dairy products that are low in fat (1½ percent milk fat or less) or fat-free. Good low-fat cheese choices include ½ percent cottage cheese; part-skim mozzarella; part-skim ricotta; Parmesan; and solid cheeses with 5 to 6 grams of fat or less per ounce. Nonfat yogurt with fruit is an excellent source of calcium that makes a refreshing snack. To replace cream cheese, you could try Neufchâtel or light cream cheese, but these are only a third less fat, so they still contain significant amounts of fat if you use generous amounts of the product.

There is a myth that margarine is lower in fat than

butter and better for you. Margarine is 100 percent fat, just like butter, and research suggests that both margarine and butter have artery-clogging properties, particularly when the first ingredient on the margarine is "hydrogenated" oil. For breakfast, you might want to consider using a teaspoon of jam or jelly on toast instead of butter or margarine. On other foods, such as potatoes or pasta, use only small amounts (one teaspoon) of low-fat margarine, or try nonfat versions of spreads, salad dressings, and sour cream.

In cooking, try to use less oil or switch to a product that has some sort of liquid polyunsaturated vegetable oil as the first ingredient. (It may be the second ingredient if water is listed first.) Ideally, you want a margarine or cooking oil with only 1 gram or less of saturated fat. Generally, the higher the polyunsaturated-to-saturated fat ratio, the better.

The dairy section also contains nondairy creamers. They may say "contains no cholesterol," which is true. However, what the front of the label does not tell you is that they are usually high in saturated fat from tropical oils, which are known to raise blood cholesterol. It is best to avoid these artificial creamers and use milk that is 1 percent or less butterfat in your coffee or tea. Some fat-free creamers may contain sugar, so they, too, should be used in moderation.

Eggs

Eggs can be a part of a healthy diet when used in moderation (fewer than three egg yolks per week). The yolk contains all of the fat and cholesterol. The white contains half the protein and none of the fat or cholesterol. In many recipes, you can replace a whole egg with two egg whites without seriously affecting the outcome of your recipe. Your grocer's freezer section will also contain several varieties of egg substitute. Try these for breakfast or in recipes to save on fat and cholesterol. No eggs are low in cholesterol, although you may hear of some marketed that way. That myth is based on a misunderstanding about how the cholesterol you eat affects the cholesterol in your bloodstream. It is still good advice to use all egg yolks in moderation if you choose to include them as a part of your healthy diet.

Inside the Perimeter

You will find some important carbohydrate sources in the interior aisles of your supermarket, but you will also encounter many processed foods loaded with saturated fat and sodium. The most important thing you can do inside the perimeter is to read the labels!

Breads, Grains, and Pastas

An important stop for shoppers interested in good taste and good nutrition is the pasta aisle. A wide variety of shapes, styles, and colors can make meals more interesting while helping you to get enough carbohydrates in your healthy diet.

The rice section also offers tasty and nutritious starchy offerings that can form the foundation of an inviting meal. Dried beans and lentils are inexpensive carbohydrates that are rich in fiber and contain some protein. If you buy canned beans, wash them for three minutes before using to remove much of the salt.

You can even make some healthy choices in the cookie and cracker section. Whole-wheat crackers with no added fat, such as Finn and Kavli, are rich in fiber and B vitamins. More manufacturers are beginning to offer nonfat cookie selections. Be aware that these tend to be high in sugar, as previously discussed, and some may also be high in sodium. Food labels can also lead you to low-fat choices such as rice cakes, low-fat popcorn, and oatmeal, while warning you of their higher-fat competitors.

Although many cereals have been fortified with vitamins and minerals, some are high in sugar, fat, and salt. Steer toward high-fiber cereals such as bran, since they will improve your digestion and may help lower your blood-glucose levels.

Fats, Oils, and Dressings

Let nutrition labels guide you through the condiments and oil shelves. Choose cooking oils such as olive and canola because they are high in monounsaturated fats, which are thought to be the healthiest for your heart. Stay away from tropical oils such as coconut and palm oil, and those containing hydrogenated fats, which may raise blood-cholesterol levels. If you choose to cook with safflower, sunflower, corn, sesame, or soybean oil, use it in moderation as well. They are not thought to raise blood cholesterol, as do the saturated fats, but remain as high in calories as any other fat. The healthiest choice to make in cooking is to use a vegetable-oil cooking spray and a non-stick pan. These will help you to make delicious, nutritious meals with only a fraction of the fat.

Many reduced-fat or nonfat salad dressings are low in fat and calories yet high in sodium. The best buy is a dressing containing less than 100 milligrams of sodium and 3 grams of fat per tablespoon. Often dressings can be diluted with water, milk, nonfat yogurt, or vinegar to reduce the sodium and/or calorie content. Look for other condiments in reduced-calorie or low-sodium versions. If you are watching your sodium intake, be very careful with mustards, pickles, soy sauces, and catsups.

Freezer Section

In the freezer section you can stock up on frozen vegetables such as corn, green peas, squash, and lima beans, which are rich in carbohydrates. In many cases, frozen vegetables actually have more vitamins than fresh vegetables that have been shipped across the country or have been allowed to sit around for several days. Of course, the healthiest choice is garden-fresh produce, but there is no significant difference between day-old and frozen produce. Frozen vegetables and fruits are far better choices than their canned versions. Canned vegetables tend to be very high in sodium and canned fruits in sugar.

The freezer section also offers many packaged dishes that can be prepared quickly but usually are laden with sodium and/or fat. You can find some low-fat entrees, although they are often high in sodium. If you choose to include these as part of your diet, you should use them with discretion. How well do they fit into your meal plan? How do they work with the other sources of fat and sodium in your diet? Remember to check the portion size to make sure that what you plan to eat matches it and the nutrient content listed.

You can check the freezer section for tasty frozen snacks and desserts, although you need to be aware of their fat content. Fruit and juice bars offer few vitamins, so don't replace all of the fruit in your diet with their frozen-dessert counterparts. Some of them contain cream or coconut and are high in fat and saturated fat.

Supermarkets stock a wide range of nonfat and low-fat frozen yogurts and low-fat ice creams. But again, these may be high in sugar. These foods should be used in moderation, and only when your blood sugar is under good control. You might find that these treats work best in your diet when you eat them after a meal rather than on their own. Monitor your blood sugar when you eat them, so that you know how your body reacts to them. Some frozen treats contain artificial sweeteners and may have less of an impact on your blood sugar than the regular low-fat versions.

Supermarkets versus Specialty Stores

Supermarkets have responded to the public interest in healthier foods by expanding their selections of low-fat and less-processed foods. Many even offer a "natural foods" section or offer specialty items traditionally found only in health food stores, such as sesame tahini, tofu, soy milk, couscous, and fruit-sweetened jam.

Health food stores also usually sell an impressive selection of grains, rice, and other dry goods in bulk, which allows you to purchase interesting and delicious foods at lower prices. They also may feature a wider range of vegetarian entrees, such as vegetarian burgers or "bacon," which can expand your food repertoire or give you new food ideas. If you do not usually shop at a health food store, you may find the experience interesting. But remember to compare food labels and prices.

Diet Supplements

New fads frequently crop up about diet supplements that make outrageous claims about their power to take off weight, boost energy, or make you live longer. Don't believe them. Since these supplements are considered neither foods nor drugs, they are not regulated by the Food and Drug Administration or the Department of Agriculture.

While stricter federal regulations have closed loopholes that allowed manufacturers to make misleading claims on food labels, you cannot be as confident about the validity of such claims on vitamin and mineral supplements. You cannot be guaranteed that their health claims are valid.

It is preferable to get minerals and vitamins through food, because they are absorbed better that way and food provides fiber, which is absent from supplements. There are also many more nutrients the body needs that are not found in pills. Taking high doses of many vitamins and minerals is known to decrease your ability to absorb them, so be cautious before you start taking megadoses (more than 200 percent of the RDA). You should always be cautious when choosing supplements. Consult your doctor or a registered dietitian for advice on whether you need supplements and, if so, which products are best.

Now that you know how to shop for healthy, low-fat foods, you can experiment with them in the delicious recipes presented in Chapter Seven.

Healthy Recipes

H ere are some recipes you can use to help build a healthy diet for you and your family. They are divided into Soups, Salads, and Appetizers; Main Dishes; Vegetables and Side Dishes; Desserts; and Muffins and Quick Breads. We have listed the calories and the number of grams of fat, protein, carbohydrate, fiber, and sodium per serving.

Most of these recipes are quick and easy to prepare, and many of them freeze well. You may find these recipes helpful when creating your "staples list" to make shopping and meal planning easier, as discussed in Chapter Six. These recipes have been developed and tested in the kitchens of the Stedman Center for Nutritional Studies restaurant, Innovations, or in the kitchens of the professional nutrition staff. We would like to extend a special recognition to John Beverly, Tim Higgins, and Patty Yunker for their significant contributions to these recipes. We hope you and your family enjoy them!

Split Pea Soup

	Vegetable cooking spray
2	cups chopped onion
1	cup diced carrot
½	cup diced celery
3	cloves garlic, minced
1	pound split peas, cleaned
¾	teaspoon salt
½	teaspoon ground black pepper
8	cups water

Coat the bottom of a large nonstick saucepan with cooking spray and sauté the onion, carrot, and celery until the onion is translucent. Add the garlic and sauté 1 minute more. Add the peas, salt, and pepper. Add the water and bring to a boil. Skim and simmer, partially covered, 3 hours, or until thick. (This soup can be made ahead of time and frozen, then thawed and reheated.)

Yield: 12 1-cup servings

Exchanges: 2 starch or 1½ starch plus 1 protein*

Since peas have some protein in them, you can be more flexible in how you use your exchanges with this recipe. It can count as either 2 starch or 1½ starch plus ½ protein.

Nutritional analysis per serving: calories 146; fat 0.5 g; protein 9.8 g; carbohydrate 26.4 g; fiber 10.5 g; sodium 151 mg.

Fruit Soup

- ½ cup dried prunes, pitted
- ½ cup dried apricot halves
- ½ cup dried pear halves
- ½ cup raisins
- 10 cups water
- 3 apples
- 1 cup sugar
- 1 cinnamon stick
- 1 tablespoon cornstarch, dissolved in ½ cup water

Put the prunes, apricots, pears, and raisins in a large saucepan, add the water, and simmer until soft. Peel and core the apples, slice, and add to the dried-fruit mixture. Add the sugar and cinnamon stick, and continue cooking until the apple is tender. Remove the pan from the heat. Using a slotted spoon, transfer the fruit to a large serving bowl. Add the cornstarch slurry to the cooking liquid and stir over low heat until the mixture is thick and clear. Pour the hot liquid over the fruit. Serve hot or cold, garnished with a dollop of Mock Sour Cream (page 104) if desired.

Yield: 12 1-cup servings

Exchanges: 2 fruit

Nutritional analysis per serving: calories 153; fat 0.3 g; protein 0.8 g; carbohydrate 40 g; fiber 3.2 g; sodium 8 mg.

White Gazpacho

4	cups water
2	cups plain nonfat yogurt
1	tablespoon cider vinegar
1	teaspoon salt
¼	teaspoon ground black pepper
3	cucumbers, peeled and chopped
3	cloves garlic, minced
1	cup diced fresh tomatoes
½	cup chopped scallions
½	cup chopped parsley
1	apple, peeled and diced

Combine all the ingredients in a large container and mix well. Cover and refrigerate at least 4 hours, or overnight. Serve cold.

Yield: 10 1-cup servings

Exchanges: 2 vegetable

Nutritional analysis per serving: calories 52; fat 0.3 g; protein 3.6 g; carbohydrate 9.6 g; fiber 1.5 g; sodium 257 mg.

South-of-the-Border Bean Dip

1   (12- or 14-ounce) can fat-free refried beans
1   (12-ounce) can white hominy, drained
¼   cup plain nonfat yogurt
½   cup salsa
1   tablespoon minced garlic

Combine all the ingredients in a large bowl and mix well. Heat in the microwave if desired. (This doubles as a bean burrito filler.)

Yield: 6 servings

Exchanges: 1½ starch plus 1 fat gram

Nutritional analysis per serving: calories 122; fat 1.3 g; protein 6 g; carbohydrate 24.2 g; fiber 7.6 g; sodium 269 mg.

Vinaigrette

1   cup vegetable broth or water
1   tablespoon cornstarch, dissolved in a small
     amount of water
1   teaspoon Dijon mustard
1   clove garlic, minced
1   teaspoon salt
½   teaspoon ground black pepper
½   cup red-wine vinegar
3   tablespoons olive oil

Heat the broth in a small saucepan until boiling. Off the heat, stir in the cornstarch slurry. Return the pan to low heat and simmer, stirring with a whisk, until the mixture thickens. Whisk together the mustard, garlic, salt, pepper, vinegar, and oil. Add to the thickened liquid and mix to combine. Allow to cool, then refrigerate.

Yield: 14 2-tablespoon servings

Exchanges: 3 fat grams

Nutritional analysis per serving: calories 42; fat 3.2 g; protein 0.5 g; carbohydrate 3.1 g; fiber 0.3 g; sodium 275 mg.

Vegetable Pasta Salad

1¾   cups pasta
1   (10-ounce) package frozen mixed
   vegetables
1   can navy beans
4   tablespoons oil-and-vinegar salad dressing

Prepare the pasta and the vegetables according to package directions. Meanwhile, rinse the beans under cold running water for 3 minutes. Add the vegetables, beans, and vinaigrette to the pasta, and toss to combine.

Yield: 8 servings

Exchanges: 2 starch plus ½ vegetable plus 5 fat grams

Nutritional analysis per serving: calories 187; fat 4.8 g; protein 7 g; carbohydrate 29.9 g; fiber 6 g; sodium 13 mg.

Cranberry-Apple Relish

2	cups fresh cranberries, cleaned
2	medium apples, peeled and diced
¼	cup frozen apple juice concentrate
2	oranges, peeled and sectioned
1	cup water
½	cup sugar

Combine all the ingredients in a large, heavy saucepan. Bring to a boil, then lower the heat, cover, and simmer 15 to 20 minutes, or until the fruit is soft. Serve warm or at room temperature.

Yield: 12 ¼-cup servings

Exchanges: 1 fruit

Nutritional analysis per serving: calories 71; fat 0.2 g; protein 0.4 g; carbohydrate 19.2 g; fiber 1.8 g; sodium 3 mg.

Mock Sour Cream

- 1 cup low-fat cottage cheese
- 2 tablespoons skim milk
- 1 tablespoon lemon juice

Put all the ingredients in a blender and process until smooth.

Yield: 8 2-tablespoon servings

Exchanges: free food

Nutritional analysis per serving: calories 22.3; fat 0.3 g; protein 3.6 g; carbohydrate 1.1 g; fiber 0 g; sodium 117 mg.

Cajun Black Beans and Rice

2	cups rice, dry
1	tablespoon olive oil
⅓	cup chopped onion
1	tablespoon minced garlic
1	teaspoon Cajun seasoning, or to taste
2	cans black beans
4	ounces shredded sharp cheddar cheese

Prepare the rice according to package directions, omitting any added fat or salt. Heat the oil in a large nonstick skillet and sauté the onion until it begins to turn translucent. Add the garlic and the Cajun seasoning, and sauté 1 minute more. Drain most of the liquid from the beans and add them to the onion mixture. Cook about 5 minutes, adding water as needed to keep the mixture from drying out. Mix in the cheese and heat until bubbling. Serve the beans over the rice.

Yield: 8 servings

Exchanges: 4 starch plus ½ protein plus 5 fat grams

Nutritional analysis per serving: calories 351; fat 5.1 g; protein 14.5 g; carbohydrate 60.3 g; fiber 3.9 g; sodium 91.6 mg.

Red Beans and Rice

1	pound dried kidney beans
5	cups water
1⅔	cups chopped celery
1⅔	cups chopped onion
1⅔	cups chopped green bell pepper
1½	teaspoons dried oregano
1	tablespoon cayenne, or to taste
1	teaspoon salt
½	teaspoon ground black pepper
2	cups rice, uncooked

Soak the beans overnight in 1½ quarts water. Drain and put them in a large, heavy pot. Add the 5 cups water, celery, onion, green pepper, oregano, cayenne, salt, and pepper. Bring to a boil and skim. Lower the heat and simmer 60 to 90 minutes, or until the beans start to fall apart. Meanwhile, prepare the rice according to package directions, omitting any added fat or salt. Serve the beans over the rice.

Yield: 10 servings

Exchanges: 3 starch plus 2 vegetable plus 1 fat gram

Nutritional analysis per serving: calories 306; fat 0.8 g; protein 14 g; carbohydrate 61.2 g; fiber 8.2 g; sodium 248 mg.

Fast Bean Burritos

1⅓ cups rice
1 teaspoon olive oil
½ cup chopped onion
1 tablespoon minced garlic
1 (12-ounce) can fat-free refried beans
1 (12-ounce) can white hominy
8 flour or corn tortillas
½ cup shredded sharp cheddar cheese
1½ cups salsa
Jalapeño chile peppers (optional)

Prepare the rice according to package directions, omitting any added fat or salt. Heat the oil in a large nonstick skillet and sauté the onion until it is translucent. Add the garlic and sauté 1 minute more. Mix in the beans and the hominy, and cook until hot. Divide the filling among the tortillas, sprinkle with cheese, wrap, and serve accompanied by salsa, rice, and jalapeño peppers, if desired.

Yield: 8 servings

Exchanges: 4 starch plus 1 vegetable plus 8 fat grams

Nutritional analysis per serving: calories 316; fat 7.8 g; protein 8.8 g; carbohydrate 54.9 g; fiber 3.7 g; sodium 339 mg.

Lentil Terrine

- 1 cup dried lentils
- 1½ teaspoons olive oil
- 1½ cups chopped onion
- 4 egg whites
- 1 teaspoon cumin seed
- ¼ teaspoon dried thyme
- ½ cup evaporated skim milk
- ½ cup plain bread crumbs
- ¼ cup chopped walnuts
- Vegetable cooking spray

Preheat the oven to 350°F. Cook the lentils according to package directions. Heat the oil in a large nonstick skillet and sauté the onion until translucent. Purée the lentils, onion, egg whites, cumin, and thyme in a food processor. Fold in the milk, bread crumbs, and walnuts. Transfer the mixture to a loaf pan coated with vegetable cooking spray. Smooth the top, cover with foil, and bake 45 minutes. Let rest 20 minutes to set. Cut into 6 slices and serve.

Yield: 6 servings

Exchanges: 2 starch plus 1 protein plus 5 fat grams

Nutritional analysis per serving: calories 227; fat 5.13 g; protein 15.2 g; carbohydrate 31 g; fiber 5.1 g; sodium 128 mg.

Quick Spinach "Lasagna"

1	(12-ounce) package pasta shells
1	(10-ounce) package frozen spinach
2	cups spaghetti sauce
1⅓	cups low-fat cottage cheese
⅓	cup grated parmesan cheese

Prepare the pasta and the spinach according to package directions. Meanwhile, heat the spaghetti sauce in a saucepan. Drain the pasta well and arrange it in a layer in a baking dish. Squeeze as much water as possible from the spinach and layer it over the pasta. Layer the cottage cheese over the spinach. Pour the sauce on top, sprinkle with the parmesan, and bake at 350°F for 25–30 minutes or until sauce is bubbly. Let dish sit for about 10 minutes before serving.

Yield: 8 servings

Exchanges: 2½ starch plus 1 vegetable plus 1 protein plus 5 fat grams

Nutritional analysis per serving: calories 277; fat 5.1 g; protein 13.7 g; carbohydrate 44.3 g; fiber 4.2 g; sodium 553 mg.

Pasta Florentine

    3   cups pasta spirals
    1   teaspoon olive oil
    1   tablespoon minced garlic
   ½   cup sliced mushrooms
    1   cup chopped fresh spinach
    3   tablespoons grated parmesan cheese
   ½   teaspoon ground black pepper, or to taste

Cook the pasta according to package directions. Meanwhile, heat the oil in a nonstick skillet and sauté the garlic. Add the mushrooms and cook until they release their juices. Transfer the mixture to a large serving bowl. Add the pasta, spinach, and cheese, season with pepper, and toss to mix.

Yield: 4 servings

Exchanges: 2 starch plus 1 vegetable plus 3 fat grams

Nutritional analysis per serving: calories 185; fat 3 g; protein 7.4 g; carbohydrate 32 g; fiber 2.4 g; sodium 84 mg.

Pasta and Peas

12	ounces pasta shells
1½	cups frozen peas
	Vegetable cooking spray
5	cups chopped onion
⅔	cup grated parmesan cheese

Prepare the pasta and the peas according to package directions. Meanwhile, coat a large nonstick skillet with vegetable cooking spray and sauté the onion until translucent and caramelized. Mix the onion, peas, and cheese into the pasta and serve immediately.

Yield: 5 servings

Exchanges: 2½ starch plus 1 protein plus 4 fat grams

Nutritional analysis per serving: calories 246; fat 4.2 g; protein 12.3 g; carbohydrate 40.4 g; fiber 5.8 g; sodium 258 mg.

Quick Chicken Dinner

- 2 cups rice
- 1 (10-ounce) package frozen mixed vegetables
- 1 cup plain bread crumbs
- ⅓ cup grated parmesan cheese
- ½ teaspoon dried oregano
- 12 ounces skinless, boneless chicken breast, cubed
- ⅓ cup skim milk

Prepare the rice and the vegetables according to package directions, omitting any added fat or salt. Meanwhile, put the bread crumbs, parmesan, and oregano in a plastic bag and shake to mix. Moisten the chicken cubes in the milk, place them in the bag with the bread crumbs, and shake to coat. Put the chicken in a microwave-safe baking dish, cover loosely with wax paper, and microwave at full power about 5 minutes, or until cooked through. Serve the chicken over the mixed rice and vegetables.

Yield: 4 servings

Exchanges: 3½ starch plus 1 vegetable plus 3 protein plus 6 fat grams

Nutritional analysis per serving: calories 457; fat 6.2 g; protein 38 g; carbohydrate 57 g; fiber 4.2 g; sodium 412 mg.

Chicken and "Dumplings"

1¼	pounds skinless, boneless chicken breast
5	cups low-sodium chicken broth
8	ounces lasagna noodles, broken up, dry weight
1	cup frozen lima beans
⅛	teaspoon ground black pepper, or to taste
2	tablespoons cornstarch, dissolved in ¼ cup cold water

Put the chicken in a microwave-safe dish with ½ cup of the chicken broth. Cover and microwave at full power 8 to 10 minutes, or until cooked through. Shred the chicken and reserve in the refrigerator. Put the chicken cooking liquid along with the rest of the broth in a large saucepan set over high heat and cook until reduced by one half. Lower the heat to a simmer and add the noodles and the lima beans. Season with pepper and cook 12 to 15 minutes, or until done. Add the cornstarch slurry and stir until thickened. Add the chicken and serve.

Yield: 8 servings

Exchanges: 2 starch plus 3 protein plus 1 fat gram

Nutritional analysis per serving: calories 291; fat 5.38 g; protein 30.5 g; carbohydrate 28 g; fiber 3.9 g; sodium 549 mg.

Crispy Chicken

¼   cup low-calorie Italian salad dressing
1¼   pounds skinless, boneless chicken breast
½   teaspoon dried rosemary
1½   tablespoons grated parmesan cheese
3½   cups cornflakes, crushed

Put the salad dressing in a glass or ceramic container and add the chicken. Cover, refrigerate, and allow to marinate 3 to 4 hours. Preheat the oven to 400°F. Mix the rosemary and cheese into the cornflakes. Remove the chicken from the marinade and toss it in the cornflake mixture to coat. Place the chicken in a baking dish, cover with foil, and cook 40 minutes. Remove foil and cook 10 minutes more to crisp.

Yield: 5 servings

Exchanges: 1 starch plus 4 protein plus 7 fat grams

Nutritional analysis per serving: calories 278; fat 6.8 g; protein 37 g; carbohydrate 14.4 g; fiber 0.4 g; sodium 373 mg.

Turkey Soft Tacos

1   pound turkey breast, ground
1   packet taco seasoning mix
1   can kidney beans
6   flour tortillas
¾   cup salsa
6   tablespoons plain nonfat yogurt
½   cup shredded sharp cheddar cheese
     Shredded lettuce
     Chopped fresh tomatoes

Mix the turkey and the taco seasoning, and microwave at full power until cooked, about 10 minutes. Meanwhile, rinse the beans in a colander under cold running water for 3 minutes. Divide the meat and beans among the tortillas. Top with 2 tablespoons salsa and 1 tablespoon yogurt, roll up, and sprinkle with cheese. Heat in the microwave. Garnish with shredded lettuce and chopped tomato before serving.

Yield: 6 servings

Exchanges: 2½ starch plus 3 protein plus 9 fat grams

Nutritional analysis per serving: calories 362; fat 9.4 g; protein 34 g; carbohydrate 36.6 g; fiber 6.9 g; sodium 285 mg.

Curried Pork Loin

- 1½   pounds pork tenderloin
- 1   clove garlic, minced
- ¼   teaspoon dried thyme
- 2   tablespoons Dijon mustard
- 2   tablespoons honey
- 2   tablespoons chopped parsley
- 1½   teaspoons curry powder
- 1   tablespoon finely chopped pecans

Preheat the oven to 450°F. Trim all visible fat from the pork loin and place it in a roasting pan. Combine the garlic, thyme, mustard, honey, parsley, and curry powder in a small bowl and whisk to mix. Spread the mixture evenly over the meat and sprinkle with the pecans. Roast 10 to 15 minutes, or until golden brown. Turn the oven down to 325°F. and continue roasting, covering with foil to prevent overbrowning if necessary. Cook to an internal temperature of 150°F. as measured on an instant-read thermometer. Let rest 15 minutes before serving.

Yield: 8 servings

Exchanges: 4 protein plus 13 fat grams

Nutritional analysis per serving: calories 261; fat 13.3 g; protein 28.4 g; carbohydrate 5.6 g; fiber 0.3 g; sodium 113 mg.

Mexican Corn Casserole

2 (10-ounce) packages frozen corn kernels
   Vegetable cooking spray
1 cup chopped onion
2 cloves garlic, minced
1 teaspoon chili powder, or to taste
½ cup chopped fresh tomatoes
1 cup chopped green bell pepper
2 tablespoons cornstarch
2 cups evaporated skim milk
1 egg, lightly beaten
⅛ teaspoon ground black pepper
½ cup shredded mozzarella cheese

Preheat the oven to 350°F. Cook the corn according to package directions. Meanwhile, coat a large nonstick skillet with vegetable cooking spray and sauté the onion until translucent. Add the garlic and chili powder and sauté 1 minute more. Add the tomato and green pepper, and cook until heated through. Set aside. Dissolve the cornstarch in ¼ cup of the milk and stir the slurry into the rest of the milk. Stir the thickened milk into the vegetable mixture, then stir in the egg. Season with pepper. Coat a large baking dish with vegetable cooking spray, fill with the mixture, and top with the cheese. Cover with foil and bake 20 minutes. Remove foil and bake 5 to 10 minutes more, or until browned.

Yield: 6 servings

Exchanges: 1 protein plus 2 starch plus 1 vegetable plus 5.4 fat grams

Nutritional analysis per serving: calories 241; fat 4.1 g; protein 16.2 g; carbohydrate 34.7 g; fiber 5 g; sodium 225 mg.

Spinach and Brown Rice Casserole

1	cup brown rice
1	(10-ounce) package frozen spinach
1	teaspoon olive oil
1	cup chopped onion
2	cups sliced mushrooms
2	cloves garlic, minced
1	egg, lightly beaten
1	tablespoon whole wheat flour
2	cups low-fat cottage cheese
¼	teaspoon dried thyme
⅛	teaspoon ground black pepper, or to taste
2	tablespoons grated parmesan cheese
	Vegetable cooking spray
2	tablespoons sunflower seeds

Preheat the oven to 375°F. Prepare the rice and the spinach according to package directions, omitting any added fat or salt. Meanwhile, heat the oil in a large non-stick skillet and sauté the onion, mushrooms, and garlic until softened. In a small bowl, mix the egg, flour, and cottage cheese, and stir it into the onion mixture in the skillet. Squeeze as much water as possible from the spinach and add it to the skillet, along with the rice, thyme, pepper, and 1 tablespoon of the cheese. Mix to combine. Transfer the mixture to a baking dish coated with spray oil. Top with the remaining 1 tablespoon cheese and the sunflower seeds. Bake 30 minutes, or until bubbling hot.

Yield: 8 servings

Exchanges: 1 starch plus 2 vegetables plus 1 protein plus 4 fat grams

Nutritional analysis per serving: calories 177; fat 3.5 g; protein 12 g; carbohydrate 24.9 g; fiber 1.9 g; sodium 288 mg.

Baked "Stuffed" Cod

2	baking potatoes
2¼	pounds cod fillets
1	tablespoon olive oil
1¼	cups chopped onion
1¼	cups sliced carrot
1¼	cups sliced celery
¼	teaspoon ground mace
¼	teaspoon curry powder
½	teaspoon salt
¼	teaspoon white pepper
	Vegetable cooking spray
1	cup evaporated skim milk

Preheat the oven to 350°F. Bake the potatoes in the microwave. When they are cool enough to handle, scoop the flesh from the peel. Cut 1 pound of the cod into cubes and purée it with the potato in a food processor. Set aside in the refrigerator. Heat the olive oil in a large nonstick skillet and sauté the onion, carrot, and celery until the onion is translucent. Add the mace, curry powder, salt, and pepper and sauté 1 minute more. Remove from the heat and set aside to cool to room temperature. Coat a large baking dish with spray oil and line the bottom with the remaining cod fillets. Combine half the vegetable mixture with the puréed cod and potato, adding milk as necessary. Spread this mixture over the fillets. Top with the remaining vegetable mixture. Cover with foil and bake 30 minutes, or until the fish is cooked; it will look slightly puffy. Serve with nonfat tartar sauce and lemon, if desired.

Yield: 8 servings

Exchanges: 1 starch plus 3 protein plus 3 fat grams

Nutritional analysis per serving: calories 207; fat 3.5 g; protein 26.3 g; carbohydrate 17 g; fiber 2.2 g; sodium 271 mg.

Baked Breaded Catfish

Vegetable cooking spray
½   cup bread crumbs, plain
½   cup flour
3   tablespoons grated parmesan cheese
¾   teaspoon paprika
⅛   teaspoon salt
⅛   teaspoon ground black pepper
1½ pounds catfish fillets
¾   cup plain low-fat yogurt

Preheat the oven to 400°F. Coat a baking pan large enough to hold all the fillets in one layer with spray oil. Combine the bread crumbs, flour, cheese, paprika, salt, and pepper in a large flat dish. Dip the fillets in the yogurt, allow the excess to drip off, then dredge in the bread-crumb mixture. Arrange the fillets in the baking pan and cook 15 minutes, or until done.

Yield: 8 servings

Exchanges: 1 starch plus 3 protein plus 4 fat grams

Nutritional analysis per serving: calories 175; fat 2.6 g; protein 24 g; carbohydrate 12.6 g; fiber 0.5 g; sodium 268 mg.

Ginger Salmon

- 2 tablespoons rice vinegar
- 1 tablespoon low-sodium soy sauce
- 1 teaspoon sesame oil
- 1 teaspoon minced ginger
- ½ teaspoon minced garlic
- 1⅛ pounds salmon fillet
  Vegetable cooking spray
- 2 tablespoons minced scallions
  Lime wedges for garnish

Combine the vinegar, soy sauce, oil, ginger, and garlic in a small bowl and whisk to mix. Place the salmon in a shallow baking dish and pour the mixture over it. Cover with plastic wrap and allow to marinate in the refrigerator 1 hour. Preheat the oven to 450°F. Coat a baking sheet with spray oil, place the fish on it, top with the remaining marinade, and cook 7 to 10 minutes, or until cooked through. Sprinkle the scallion over the fish and garnish with lime wedges.

Yield: serves 6

Exchanges: 2 protein plus 3.5 fat grams

Nutritional analysis per serving: calories 133; fat 3.7 g; protein 17.1 g; carbohydrate 1.2 g; fiber 0 g; sodium 138 mg.

Asparagus and Shiitake Mushroom Stir-Fry

1	pound asparagus
2	ounces shiitake mushrooms
1	teaspoon olive oil
⅛	teaspoon salt
¼	teaspoon ground black pepper
⅛	teaspoon ground coriander, or to taste

Wash the asparagus and trim ¼ inch from the bottom of each stalk. Using a vegetable peeler, peel the stalks to just below the tip. Cut the asparagus on the diagonal into ½-inch slices. Quickly rinse and dry the mushrooms, remove the stems, and cut into ¼-inch slices. Heat the oil in a large nonstick skillet. Stir-fry the asparagus 2 minutes. Add 2 tablespoons water, cover, and cook 3 minutes more. Add the mushrooms and cook, uncovered, 2 minutes, or until done. Season with salt, pepper, and coriander, and serve immediately.

Yield: 5 servings

Exchanges: 2 vegetable plus 3 fat grams

Nutritional analysis per serving: calories 54; fat 2.9 g; protein 2.2 g; carbohydrate 6.4 g; fiber 3 g; sodium 5 mg.

Almond Green Beans

- 1 pound green beans
- 2 tablespoons slivered almonds
- 1 teaspoon sesame oil
- ¼ teaspoon ground black pepper

Wash and trim the green beans, put them in a microwave-safe dish, sprinkle with water, cover, and microwave at full power 6 to 8 minutes, or until tender. Meanwhile, toast the almonds in a small nonstick skillet until golden. Drain the green beans and toss with the sesame oil, almonds, and pepper.

Yield: 5 servings

Exchanges: 2 vegetable plus 3 fat grams

Nutritional analysis per serving: calories 54; fat 2.9 g; protein 2.2 g; carbohydrate 6.4 g; fiber 3 g; sodium 5 mg.

Honey-Glazed Carrots

1	pound baby carrots
¼	cup water
3	teaspoons honey
1	tablespoon Dijon mustard
1	tablespoon cider vinegar

Put all the ingredients in a saucepan and bring to a boil. Lower the heat and simmer 15 to 20 minutes, or until the carrots are tender.

Yield: 5 servings

Exchanges: 1 vegetable plus ½ fruit

Nutritional analysis per serving: calories 50; fat 0.6 g; protein 0.9 g; carbohydrate 11.3 g; fiber 0.1 g; sodium 70 mg.

Roasted Red Potatoes

2   pounds red new potatoes
Vegetable cooking spray
1   teaspoon ground black pepper

Preheat the oven to 450°F. Scrub the potatoes, dry them well, and cut them into wedges. Arrange the wedges on a baking sheet and coat with spray oil. Bake 15 minutes. Spray with oil again and sprinkle with pepper. Bake 15 minutes more, or until browned.

Yield: 4 servings

Exchanges: 2 starch

Nutritional analysis per serving: calories 135.9; fat 0.2 g; protein 3.6 g; carbohydrate 31 g; fiber 2.9 g; sodium 10 mg.

Mashed Potatoes

1½   pounds all-purpose potatoes
¼   cup buttermilk
¼   teaspoon salt

Peel the potatoes and cut them into 1-inch chunks. Place them in a saucepan and add water to cover. Bring to a boil and cook until soft. Drain, reserving the cooking liquid. Add the buttermilk and salt, and mash the potatoes with a fork or a potato masher, adding enough of the reserved cooking liquid to reach the desired consistency. Reheat in the microwave if necessary.

Yield: 6 ½-cup servings

Exchanges: 1 starch

Nutritional analysis per serving: calories 71.4; fat 0.2 g; protein 2.1 g; carbohydrate 15.8 g; fiber 1.4 g; sodium 105 mg.

Potato Pancakes

1	pound all-purpose potatoes
2	cups diced onion
¾	cup diced red bell pepper
4	egg whites
½	teaspoon salt
1	teaspoon ground black pepper

Put the potatoes in a saucepan, add water to cover, and cook about 10 minutes. When the potatoes are cool enough to handle, peel and grate them. Mix the grated potatoes with the onion, red pepper, egg whites, salt, and pepper. Preheat the oven to 350°F. Form the potato mixture into 8 pancakes. Coat a nonstick skillet with spray oil, heat, and brown the pancakes on both sides. Transfer the pancakes to a cookie sheet and bake 10 to 15 minutes, or until done. Serve with Mock Sour Cream (page 104).

Yield: 8 pancakes, 1 per serving

Exchanges: 1 starch

Nutritional analysis per serving: calories 77; fat 0.1 g; protein 3.4 g; carbohydrate 15.8 g; fiber 1.7 g; sodium 164 mg.

Apple-Apricot Stuffing

1   teaspoon peanut oil
2   cups chopped onion
3   cups sliced mushrooms
2   cups chopped celery
1   medium apple, peeled and diced
¼   cup dried apricot halves
1   cup vegetable broth or water
5   cups fresh bread cubes
¼   cup chopped pecans
¼   teaspoon ground sage
½   teaspoon ground thyme
½   teaspoon ground black pepper
    Vegetable cooking spray

Preheat the oven to 325°F. Heat the oil in a large, heavy nonstick saucepan. Sauté the onion, mushroom, and celery until the onion is translucent. Add the apples and apricots, and cook a few minutes more. Add the stock and bring to a boil. Remove from the heat and mix in the bread cubes, pecans, sage, thyme, and pepper. Coat a 10 × 10-inch baking pan with spray oil. Transfer the mixture to the pan, cover with foil, and bake 30 minutes. Remove the foil and bake 10 minutes more.

Yield: 8 1-cup servings

Exchanges: 1 starch plus 1 vegetable plus 3 fat grams

Nutritional analysis per serving: calories 122; fat 3.2 g; protein 3.4 g; carbohydrate 21.4 g; fiber 3.4 g; sodium 301 mg.

Apple Cobbler

You can also make this with blueberries (2 pints fresh or a 24-ounce bag frozen) or peaches.

6	cups apple slices
4	tablespoons white flour
5	tablespoons sugar
2	tablespoons orange juice
1	tablespoon grated orange zest
1	cup whole wheat flour
1	teaspoon baking powder
½	teaspoon baking soda
1	tablespoon canola oil
½	cup buttermilk
	Vegetable cooking spray

Preheat the oven to 375°F. Put the apples, 3 tablespoons of the white flour, 4 tablespoons of the sugar, and the orange juice and zest in a large saucepan. Bring to a boil, then remove from the heat and set aside to cool. Put the whole wheat flour, the remaining 1 tablespoon white flour, the remaining 1 tablespoon sugar, and the baking powder and baking soda in a bowl and mix to combine. In another bowl, whisk the canola oil into the buttermilk. Add this to the flour mixture and mix to make a soft dough. Coat a baking dish with spray oil, layer the apple mixture in it, and top with the flour mixture. Bake until browned.

Yield: 8 ½-cup servings

Exchanges: 1 starch plus 1 fruit plus 2.5 fat grams

Nutritional analysis per serving: calories 165; fat 2.41 g; protein 3 g; carbohydrate 34 g; fiber 4 g; sodium 110 mg.

Bananas Baked in Filo with Chocolate Sauce

3 ounces dark chocolate
4 bananas
4 sheets filo dough
Vegetable cooking spray

Preheat the oven to 400°F. Melt the chocolate in the microwave. Meanwhile, peel the bananas and split them. Cut the sheets of filo in half to form 8 rectangles. Lay out one of the half-sheets on a work surface and coat with spray oil. Drizzle 2 teaspoons of the melted chocolate in a line near the far end, place a banana half in the center of the rectangle on top of it, and begin rolling up the filo toward you. After two turns, tuck in the sides of the filo; then continue rolling. Place on a nonstick baking sheet, and repeat the process with the other filo sheets and bananas. Bake 10 minutes, or until the dough just begins to brown. Serve hot or cold, topped with 1 teaspoon melted chocolate.

Yield: 8 servings

Exchanges: 2 fruit plus 2 fat grams

Nutritional analysis per serving: calories 113; fat 2 g; protein 1.6 g; carbohydrate 22 g; fiber 1.3 g; sodium 39 mg.

Poached Pears

4	cups water
½	cup sugar
1	stick cinnamon
3	pears
1	tablespoon lemon juice
3	tablespoons orange juice

Combine the water, sugar, and cinnamon stick in a stainless steel saucepan and bring to a boil. Meanwhile, peel the pears, cut them in half, and remove the core. Coat each pear half with lemon juice as you work to prevent it from discoloring. When the sugar syrup is boiling, reduce the heat, add the pears, lemon juice, and orange juice, and simmer 20 to 30 minutes, or until the pears are tender when pierced with a knife. Remove the pears from the syrup with a slotted spoon. When they are cool enough to handle, make five or six vertical slices in the thick end of each pear half to within 1 inch of the stem end, and fan out the slices. Serve warm or cold. If desired, top with 1 tablespoon Raspberry Sauce (page 136).

Yield: 6 servings

Exchanges: 1 fruit

Nutritional analysis per serving: calories 96.4; fat 0.3 g; protein 0.4 g; carbohydrate 24.4 g; fiber 2.8 g; sodium 0.3 mg.

Raspberry Sauce

1½   cups frozen raspberries, thawed
1   tablespoon grated orange zest
¼   cup vanilla low-fat yogurt

Purée the raspberries in a food processer and strain to remove the seeds. Mix in the orange zest and yogurt. If desired, sweeten with a little sugar or a nonnutritive sweetener.

Yield: 12 1-tablespoon servings

Exchanges: ½ fruit

Nutritional analysis per serving: calories 36; fat 0.1 g; protein 0.5 g; carbohydrate 9 g; fiber 1.4 g; sodium 3 mg.

Molasses Cookies

1	scant cup flour, plus more for dusting
1⅔	cups rolled oats
1	teaspoon baking soda
½	teaspoon ground cinnamon
¼	teaspoon ground ginger
⅛	teaspoon ground cloves
3	egg whites
⅔	cup sugar, plus more for dusting
3	tablespoons blackstrap molasses
⅓	cup peanut oil
2	tablespoons frozen apple juice concentrate
	Vegetable cooking spray

In a mixing bowl, combine the flour, oats, baking soda, cinnamon, ginger, and cloves, and set aside. In the bowl of an electric mixer, put the egg whites, sugar, molasses, oil, and apple juice concentrate, and mix well. Add the dry ingredients to the wet ones and beat until the batter is moist. Cover with plastic wrap and refrigerate 1 hour. Preheat the oven to 350°F. Prepare cookie sheets by coating with spray oil and dusting with flour. Make 24 cookies by rolling rounded tablespoonfuls of batter into balls, rolling them in sugar, and pressing them flat with a jar lid that has been coated with spray and dusted with sugar. Bake 8 to 10 minutes, or until done.

Yield: 24 servings

Exchanges: 1 starch plus 3.5 fat grams

Nutritional analysis per serving: calories 99.3; fat 3.4 g; protein 1.9 g; carbohydrate 15.6 g; fiber 0.6 g; sodium 62 mg.

Pumpkin Cheesecake

Vegetable cooking spray
1½ cups graham cracker crumbs
⅓ cup frozen apple juice concentrate, thawed
8 ounces part-skim ricotta cheese
1⅓ cups white sugar
¼ cup brown sugar
1¾ cups canned pumpkin purée
⅔ cup evaporated skim milk
2 tablespoons cornstarch
2 eggs
2 cups low-fat vanilla yogurt

First, make the crust. Coat a 9-inch pie plate with spray oil. Moisten the cracker crumbs with apple juice concentrate and press the mixture into the pan. Set aside. Now, make the filling. Preheat the oven to 350°F. Put the ricotta, 1 cup of the white sugar, the brown sugar, pumpkin, milk, cornstarch, eggs, and 1 cup of the yogurt in a blender and process until smooth. Pour the mixture into the prepared pie shell and bake 25 to 35 minutes, or until set around the edges but still wobbly in the center. Mix the remaining 1 cup yogurt with the remaining ⅓ cup white sugar and pour it over the top of the cheesecake, leaving a 1-inch rim around the edge. Bake 3 to 5 minutes more, or until the topping is set. Allow to cool, then refrigerate at least 4 hours. Serve cold.

Yield: 16 servings

Exchanges: 1 starch plus 2 fruit plus 3 fat grams

Nutritional analysis per serving: calories 189; fat 2.9 g; protein 5.3 g; carbohydrate 36.3 g; fiber 1 g; sodium 107 mg.

Apricot-Orange Muffins

	Vegetable cooking spray
1	cup buttermilk
½	cup brown sugar
1	egg
2	egg whites
1½	teaspoons vanilla extract
½	teaspoon almond extract
2	tablespoons grated orange zest
1	cup dried apricot halves, chopped
1½	cups white flour
1	cup whole wheat flour
1½	teaspoons baking powder
1	teaspoon baking soda
½	teaspoon salt

Preheat the oven to 350°F. and coat 12 muffin tins with spray oil. In a small bowl, combine the buttermilk, brown sugar, egg, egg whites, vanilla, almond extract, and zest, and whisk to mix. Stir in the apricots and let stand 5 minutes. Meanwhile, in a large bowl combine the white flour, whole wheat flour, baking powder, baking soda, and salt. Pour the wet ingredients into the dry ones and mix just to combine; do not overmix. Immediately divide the batter among the prepared muffin tins. Bake 35 minutes, or until done.

Yield: 12 muffins

Exchanges: 2 starch plus 1 fat gram

Nutritional analysis per serving: calories 157; fat 0.9 g; protein 5.1 g; carbohydrate 33.3 g; fiber 2.8 g; sodium 278 mg.

Lemon Muffins

	Vegetable cooking spray
3	tablespoons margarine, melted and cooled
1	egg
1	tablespoon lemon juice
1	tablespoon grated lemon zest
1	teaspoon lemon extract
1¾	cups flour
1	teaspoon baking powder
1	teaspoon baking soda
¾	cup sugar

Preheat the oven to 350°F. and coat 12 muffin tins with spray oil. In a small bowl, combine the margarine, egg, lemon juice, zest, and extract. In a large bowl, combine the flour, baking powder, baking soda, and sugar. Pour the wet ingredients into the dry ones and mix just to combine; do not overmix. Immediately divide the batter among the prepared muffin tins. Bake 12 minutes, or until done.

Yield: 12 servings

Exchanges: 2 starch plus 3.5 fat grams

Nutritional analysis per serving: calories 146; fat 3.4 g; protein 2.4 g; carbohydrate 26.8 g; fiber 0.1 g; sodium 173 mg.

Pumpkin Sunflower-Seed Bread

Vegetable cooking spray
¾ cup pumpkin purée, canned
2 tablespoons corn oil
1 egg
2 tablespoons applesauce
¼ cup sunflower seeds
1½ cups flour
1 cup sugar
1 teaspoon baking soda
¼ teaspoon ground cinnamon
¼ teaspoon ground ginger
¼ teaspoon ground allspice

Preheat the oven to 325°F. and coat a loaf pan with spray oil. In a small bowl, combine the pumpkin, oil, egg, applesauce, and sunflower seeds. In a large bowl, combine the flour, sugar, baking soda, cinnamon, ginger, and allspice. Pour the wet ingredients into the dry ones and mix just to combine; do not overmix. Immediately transfer the batter to the prepared pan. Bake 55 minutes, or until done.

Yield: 14 servings

Exchanges: 2 starch plus 3 fat grams

Nutritional analysis per serving: calories 140.2; fat 3.1 g; protein 2.2 g; carbohydrate 26.4 g; fiber 0.6 g; sodium 95 mg.

Whole Wheat Sesame Bread

Vegetable cooking spray
2 cups whole wheat flour
1 cup white flour
¼ cup toasted sesame seeds
6 tablespoons sugar
2 teaspoons baking soda
1 teaspoon salt
2 cups buttermilk

Preheat the oven to 350°F. and coat a loaf pan with spray oil. In a large bowl, combine the whole wheat flour, white flour, sesame seeds, sugar, baking soda, and salt. Add the buttermilk and mix just to combine; do not overmix. Immediately transfer the batter to the prepared pan. Bake 55 minutes, or until done.

Yield: 12 servings

Exchanges: 1½ starch plus 2 fat grams

Nutritional analysis per serving: calories 164.1; fat 2.3 g; protein 5.7 g; carbohydrate 31.5 g; fiber 3.3 g; sodium 433 mg.

Zucchini Bread

     Vegetable cooking spray
 ¼   cup apple juice
 ¼   cup skim milk
 3   scant tablespoons plain nonfat yogurt
 ½   teaspoon canola oil
 2   egg whites
 1   cup shredded zucchini
1¼   cups whole wheat flour
 ½   cup oat bran
 2   tablespoons sugar
 1   tablespoon baking powder
 ½   teaspoon baking soda
1¼   teaspoons ground cinnamon

Preheat the oven to 325°F. and coat a loaf pan with spray oil. In a medium bowl, combine the apple juice, milk, yogurt, oil, and egg whites, and whisk to mix. Stir in the shredded zucchini. In a large bowl, combine the flour, oat bran, sugar, baking powder, baking soda, and cinnamon. Pour the wet ingredients into the dry ones and mix just to combine; do not overmix. Immediately transfer the batter to the prepared pan. Bake 35 minutes, or until done.

Yield: 12 servings

Exchanges: 1 starch plus 1 fat gram

Nutritional analysis per serving: calories 74.4; fat 0.8 g; protein 3.6 g; carbohydrate 16 g; fiber 2.5 g; sodium 159 mg.

Chapter Eight

Managing Diabetes Away from Home

Eating away from home no longer means taking a vacation from healthy eating, nor does diabetes mean never dining out. Restaurants and airlines are responding to the public desire for healthier foods by offering low-fat entrees, more vegetables, and skim milk, which will help you with your needs. You can also find healthy foods at grocery stores and delicatessens when you are traveling. Eating well-balanced, low-fat meals away from home that fit into your meal plan is possible with a little planning.

On the Road

Americans' interest in eating a healthy diet has prompted fast-food chains to offer lower-fat, healthier alternatives to their traditional fare. Look for baked potatoes instead of french fries, grilled chicken sandwiches instead of breaded and fried ones, and salad bars with low-fat and nonfat dressings. Some restaurants even offer side orders of vegetables, rice, or beans.

Although many fast-food restaurants and other dining establishments offer low-fat food selections, don't forget that the best source for healthy foods while away from home is the best source for healthy foods at home—the supermarket. Just as most interstate highway exits boast a flock of fast-food restaurants or roadside diners, many exits also lead to a nearby shopping center that houses a supermarket. Many supermarkets now sell meals-to-go and single servings of fresh foods.

The simplest low-fat, food-to-go choices include fruit or single-serving nonfat or low-fat yogurts. But many supermarkets also feature extensive delicatessens and bakeries that prepare sandwiches and salads to go. A turkey sandwich is one popular low-fat offering you can probably find here. Shrimp salad is another. Make sure you ask what is in them or request your salad or sandwich be made fresh with nonfat mayonnaise. Don't forget that most of the fat and saturated fat in deli foods comes from added mayonnaise and cheese.

In the Air

If you are flying to your destination, take advantage of your airline's offer to provide special meals for customers. Call the airline at least 24 hours in advance of your scheduled flight and request the low-fat or vegetarian meal. You can also request a low-sodium meal if desired. If you have to choose one or the other, you'll probably do better by ordering a low-fat or vegetarian meal, as these are often moderate in sodium as well. Select skim milk or juice, as it fits into your meal plan, or diet soda instead of alcohol or regular soda with your meal or during the beverage service. Carry portable items such as low-fat crackers or fruit with you on the plane so you'll have a healthy snack available.

At Your Destination

Once you arrive at your vacation or business destination, try choosing accommodations with some food facilities, such as a kitchenette or a motel room with a small refrigerator, to increase your dining options and cut food costs. Ask the proprietor or other people who live in the area where you can find good supermarkets and restaurants as well as specialty food stores. Sampling local culinary specialties is one of the pleasures of travel. If you're in Maine, for instance, sample lobster; if you discover a unique bakery, try its whole wheat bread. A roadside produce market is a wonderful place to stock up on locally grown fruits and vegetables. Many cities as well as rural areas now feature weekly farmers' markets where you can sample the regional fare along with local produce.

If you're staying at a condominium or cottage with a well-equipped kitchen, bring a few simple ingredients and cooking utensils so you can cook meals there. Stock up on fresh vegetables and easy-to-prepare grains such as rice or pasta so that you'll have the makings for a healthy, low-fat meal on hand. Fresh fruit and nonfat yogurt (frozen or regular) provide tasty, simple snacks. If you get into a pinch and have no other alternative when you are traveling, instant breakfast drinks made with skim milk are a simple and nutritious breakfast or snack option.

Dining Out

As a nation, we dine out a lot. It is estimated that between 50 percent and 75 percent of all meals are eaten away from home. Often these meals are from fast-food restaurants, which rarely include fruits and vegetables on their menus. Although dining out frequently can pose difficult challenges for meeting healthy-eating guidelines, there are steps you can take to make your meals away from home as healthy as possible. You can dine out and still manage your diabetes, but it takes planning.

It is important to stick with your basic meal plan even when traveling or on holidays. Remember to be consistent. If you cut back slightly on your fat intake at breakfast, lunch, and snacks, you may be able to order a higher-fat meal choice at dinner. However, this may have an adverse effect on your blood glucose, so you need to monitor it to make sure your glucose control is not being affected.

If you dine out more than four or five times a week, restaurant meals probably are affecting your glucose control and your risk for heart disease, high blood pressure, and complications of diabetes. That's why it is important to know how to make the healthiest choices at restaurants. Dining out frequently can be a real challenge to your nutritional health for several reasons. Here are some solutions for meeting those challenges.

Most restaurants serve portions much larger than anyone needs to eat. You have several options. You could just eat what you need and leave the rest, but many people find that difficult to do. You could ask for a smaller portion. You could ask for an additional plate, putting only the amount of food you are going to eat on that plate. You could share an entree with someone else. You could ask for a take-home container at the start of the meal and remove the excess food before you start to eat.

But probably the best tool to avoid overeating in a restaurant is to be familiar with portion sizes. Take some time each month to actually measure out foods so that you are familiar with what a serving is by sight alone. If you have three exchanges of starch at dinner and wish to eat those as pasta, then measure out 1½ cups of pasta to see what that looks like on a plate. Don't be surprised if a restaurant serves 6 cups of pasta as an entree. Hardly anyone, regardless of whether or not he has diabetes, should eat that much food at a single meal.

Restaurant meals also tend to be high in fat. It is not unusual for restaurant meals to have 40 percent, 50 percent, or even greater amounts of calories coming from fat—way above the national health goal of a total of 30 percent of daily calories coming from fat. Your best defense against too much fat is to be assertive. Ask questions and make special requests of your waiter or waitress: Which dressings and sauces are low in fat? Can dressings and sauces be served on the side? Can you use lemon instead of oil as a seasoning? What are foods sautéed in? Can they be cooked in broth, wine, or water with just a hint of fat instead? Is fat trimmed from the meat? What cut is the meat? Is the skin removed from poultry dishes, and is the meat all white meat?

If your meal comes to you and is not what you ordered, then *send it back*. Remember, you are the customer and you are paying for more than just food: you are paying for service.

Restaurant food is generally high in sodium. Most restaurants will serve you a meal with more than 1,000 to 1,500 milligrams of sodium, regardless of whether they feature fast food, elegant dining, or ethnic specialties. That one meal out gives you more than one-third of your daily intake of the recommended 3,300 milligrams of sodium. If you have hypertension and are limiting your sodium to about 2,200 milligrams daily, a single restaurant meal will give you more than half of your day's intake of sodium.

Sodium comes from table salt, soy sauce, additives (such as monosodium glutamate), and natural sources of sodium in foods, such as cheese and tomatoes. You can ask to have salt withheld during preparation and not use salt at the table, but restaurants often use prepared ingredients. In general, the more processing a food has gone through, the higher the sodium content. Meals from fast-food restaurants are particularly high in sodium. You can opt for a salad rather than a cooked dish to avoid excess salt (don't forget to ask for low-fat dressing).

You may be able to balance your sodium intake by choosing lower-sodium foods at other meals, but if you dine out frequently, then too much sodium is likely to be a problem.

Finally, we all naturally tend to forget healthy-food guidelines when we dine out. Some may view dining out as a special occasion or a vacation from sensible eating. When you have diabetes and you dine out, you still need to choose foods wisely. This is never more important than when you dine out frequently.

Remember your health goals when you dine out. Eating out is not a vacation from taking care of yourself, so focus on more than just the food. Focus on the company, the atmosphere, and the luxury of not having to prepare food or clean up afterward. Follow your guideline to success with diabetes: consistency. Eat about the same amounts of the same types of foods at about the same times.

Enjoying Ethnic Foods

Many ethnic cuisines offer delicious alternatives to traditional American fare. Perhaps the lowest-fat choice is Japanese (except for tempura), but it is also very foreign to many American taste buds. Chinese food has been embraced by our hearty American appetites, but much of the food served in Chinese restaurants is loaded with sodium and fat. Look for steamed dishes and always request no MSG at these restaurants. Also avoid the many fried dishes and dishes with peanuts or other nuts. Vietnamese restaurants offer a wide range of dishes that feature seafood or vegetables that are steamed—a healthier alternative to heavier sauces or fried dishes.

Middle Eastern restaurants emphasize unusual and wholesome grain dishes that use different spices. Many Middle Eastern foods, such as hummus, baba ganoush, tabouli, and falafel, however, are very high in fat. Ask your waiter or waitress how the foods are prepared. At Indian restaurants tandoori-style meats are the lowest-fat options. Indian restaurants also offer many vegetable dishes, but these are generally made with oil, so they also tend to be high in fat.

Italian, Spanish, and Mexican restaurants center meals around nutritious carbohydrates such as pasta and beans. At these restaurants you need to watch out for cheese and cheese sauces, sour cream, and guacamole. Choose pasta primavera over spaghetti and meatballs, for instance, because the former features vegetables instead of beef. When you order beans, order whole black or pinto beans instead of refried beans, as the latter are usually made with added fat. Make sure to ask if beans are cooked with fat or bacon or pork, which might steer you to other choices on the menu. Guacamole, although very rich in monounsaturated fats, is practically all fat and very high in calories. As at any restaurant, read the menu carefully and ask your waiter or waitress to recommend or explain dishes to you. Many restaurants can make some changes to create a healthier meal for you, so work with them to get what you want.

How to Interpret Menus

Now that we have discussed the problems with restaurant dining and some tips for enjoying healthful meals out, let's look for clues that menus offer about their foods.

Question-and-Answer Menu Game

There are some words you should seek out and some words you should avoid when dining out. Here are some words you might see on a restaurant menu:

CASSEROLE	CRISPY	AU GRATIN	POACHED	CREAMED
MARINATED	FRIED	BROILED	STEAMED	BAKED
HOLLANDAISE	BOILED	GRAVY	ROASTED	AU JUS
IN ITS OWN JUICE	TOMATO JUICE	BUTTERED	PARMESAN	GRILLED

1. Five of these words indicate a food *is* high in fat. Do you know which ones they are?
2. Six of these words tell you a food *might* be high in fat. Do you know which ones they are?
3. Ten of these words tell you a food *could* be low in fat, but you may still need to ask the wait staff some questions. Can you identify them?

ANSWERS:

1. FRIED, HOLLANDAISE, AU GRATIN, GRAVY, and CREAMED. These terms all mean that the food will be high in fat. It is unlikely the chef will be able to do anything to reduce the fat content. Avoid foods described with these words.
2. CASSEROLE, MARINATED, CRISPY, BUTTERED, PARMESAN, and GRAVY. When you see these words, ask your waiter or waitress for more information, because these foods may or may not be healthy. For many of them, the chef might be able to make some modifications in the kitchen to make these foods healthier for you.
3. IN ITS OWN JUICE, BOILED, TOMATO JUICE, BROILED, POACHED, STEAMED, ROASTED, BAKED, AU JUS, and GRILLED. These words tell you a food could be prepared with little added fat, but you should always check with your waiter or waitress

anyway, just to be sure that little or no fat has been added.

Look for restaurants that give you some control over the foods you order. Choose restaurants where you can order items without their sauces and cheese, and those that offer fresh vegetables and fruits. Most fast-food restaurants now have posters or brochures that list the nutritional contents of their foods. Use these to make the healthiest choices. But remember, if you eat out frequently, sodium will be a problem. You will need to eat less sodium during the rest of the day to balance your intake. When you eat at fast-food restaurants, seek out the lower-fat selections. Look at other options for dining out if you need to eat away from home frequently.

Tips for Staying Healthy While Dining Out

- Plan ahead. Try to choose establishments that you know offer appropriate choices. Watch out for the restaurants that offer only high-calorie, low-nutrient selections, and stay away from all-you-can-eat buffets.

  Before you go into a restaurant or look at a menu, decide what kind of food you desire and how it fits into your meal plan. Don't go into a restaurant ravenous: you will be tempted to overeat. If you are so hungry that you are starving or feel light-headed or dizzy, then you are probably experiencing hypoglycemia. Monitor your blood glucose. You may need to eat something to raise your blood glucose before you go out. Eat a good source of carbohydrate, like orange juice or a piece of fruit or bread before you leave home.

- Follow your meal plan. Your meal plan is a guide to follow every day for healthful eating. If you know you are going to eat out, incorporate that day's exchanges into your meal plan. Try to eat consistently.
- Balance your choices. If you know you are going to have a dinner that is higher in fat, then eat lean the rest of the day to keep your total day's fat intake within your fat-gram budget. But don't make radical changes in your fat intake, since it could influence your blood-glucose management. Eating low-fat meals most of the time and then a dinner that is high in fat may cause your two-hour post-meal blood glucose to be high. Some people even find that their morning blood glucose is high after a high-fat dinner the night before.
- Choose low-fat foods. Choose your menu selections wisely. Look for clues that a food is low in fat, and then ask your waiter or waitress questions to find out what kind and how much fat is used in preparing dishes.
- Be moderate. Watch your portions. Remember that what you are served in a restaurant is rarely a reasonable portion. Don't overindulge just because you are dining out. If you order an appetizer, choose a nutritious one such as raw vegetables, fruit, or steamed mussels. Avoid fried appetizers or ones with heavy sauces. Remember that a couple of appetizers can make up a meal in themselves, so don't eat your dinner twice.
- Even though the salad bar sounds like a healthy, low-calorie stop, it is a minefield of calories and fat. Most offer fatty dressings, and some serve pepperoni, bacon bits, hard-boiled eggs, high-calorie soups, and even puddings or other desserts. Stick to the vegetables and choose the low-fat dressing.

- Go easy on alcohol. Be cautious about your alcohol consumption, which may be more difficult when wine is served with dinner. Alcohol is full of empty calories, and it may affect your blood glucose. If keeping tight control over your blood glucose is difficult for you, then avoid alcohol. If you can manage your glucose well, then drink in moderation when you choose alcoholic beverages. The Stedman Center and ADA recommend moderate consumption of alcohol only if your blood glucose is under control. Speak with your physician before including alcohol in your meal plan.
- Watch how often you eat out. Eating out too often can pose problems no matter how much you know about foods. Restaurant foods usually aren't prepared as healthfully as many home-cooked foods. Unless you find a truly special restaurant that serves special foods, try to limit dining out to about a couple of times a week.

Not only can you live with diabetes, you can live well. You can avoid or minimize complications of the disease by eating a healthy, balanced diet, exercising, and maintaining good glucose control. You can lose weight and reduce your blood-fat levels, along with your risk for cardiovascular disease. Most likely, you can reduce or even eliminate your medication. Most important, the suggestions in this book will enable you to be healthier than even before you were diagnosed with diabetes. Good luck and bon appétit!

Resources and Further Reading

Additional information and advice can be obtained from the following sources:

American Diabetes Association, 1660 Duke Street, Alexandria, VA 22314, 1-800-232-3472.

American Dietetic Association, 216 W. Jackson Boulevard, Suite 800, Chicago, IL 60606, 1-800-877-1600 (general information), 1-800-366-1665 (hotline).

American Heart Association, 1-800-527-6941.

Diabetes: A Guide to Living Well, by E. Lowe and G. Arsham, published in 1989 by the Diabetes Center, Wayzata, MN.

The Human Side of Diabetes, by M. Raymond, published in 1992 by Noble Press, Chicago.

Learning to Live Well with Diabetes, by M. J. Franz et al., published in 1991 by DCI Publishing, Minneapolis.

Managing Diabetes on a Budget, published in 1995 by the American Diabetes Association, Alexandria, VA.

National Heart, Lung and Blood Institute, 1-800-575-9335.

Outsmarting Diabetes, by R. S. Beaser, published in 1994 by Chronimed Publishing, Minneapolis.

Psyching Out Diabetes, by R. R. Rubin, J. Biermann, and B. Toohey, published in 1993 by Lowell House, Los Angeles.

General Index

Recipe Index

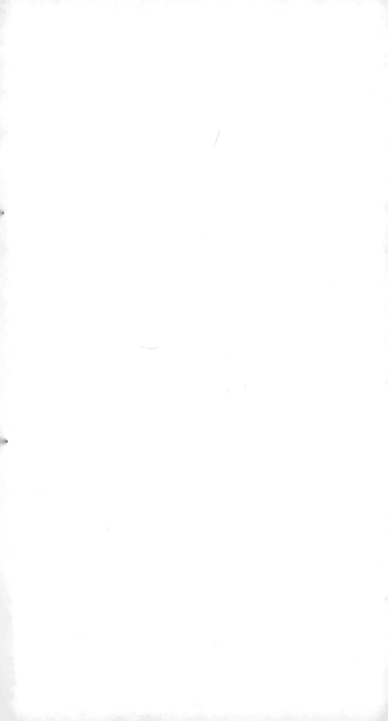